Molecular Diagnostics - Current Approaches and Their Clinical Applications

Edited by Gisela Gaina

Published in London, United Kingdom

Molecular Diagnostics - Current Approaches and Their Clinical Applications
http://dx.doi.org/10.5772/intechopen.1006439
Edited by Gisela Gaina

Contributors
Alka Shukla, Ana Karina Chávez-Escamilla, Brenda Leticia Escobedo-Guajardo, Carlos Alberto González-Villarreal, Diego José Gomes de Paula, Gabi Hewer, Genoveva Alvarez-Ojeda, Gisela Gaina, Gopal Nath, Jennifer Vieira Gomes, Juan Francisco Lugo-Ibarra, Kelly Andrewartha, Kirsty Smith, Louise Causer, Mark Shephard, María Guadalupe Moreno-Treviño, Rebecca Guy, Santiago Saavedra-Alonso, Susan Matthews, Suzana Pinheiro de Oliveira Ribeiro, Tatiana de Almeida Simão

First published in London, United Kingdom, 2025 by IntechOpen
IntechOpen is the global imprint of INTECHOPEN LIMITED, registered in England and Wales, registration number: 11086078, 167-169 Great Portland Street, London, W1W 5PF, United Kingdom

For EU product safety concerns: IN TECH d.o.o., Prolaz Marije Krucifikse Kozulić 3, 51000 Rijeka, Croatia, info@intechopen.com or visit our website at intechopen.com.

British Library Cataloguing-in-Publication Data
A catalogue record for this book is available from the British Library

Molecular Diagnostics - Current Approaches and Their Clinical Applications
Edited by Gisela Gaina
p. cm.
Print ISBN 978-1-83635-049-1
Online ISBN 978-1-83635-048-4
eBook (PDF) ISBN 978-1-83635-050-7

If disposing of this product, please recycle the paper responsibly.

Meet the editor

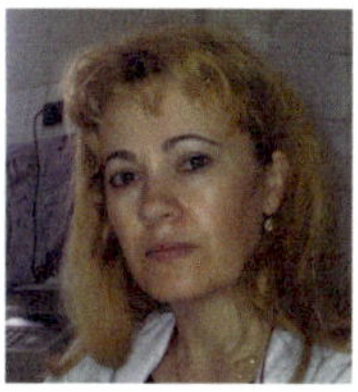

Gisela Gaina, Ph.D., currently works at 'Victor Babes" National Institute of Pathology, Bucharest, Romania. She received her Ph.D. in Biology from the University of Bucharest, Romania, in 2009, with a thesis based on the study of the proteins involved in muscular dystrophies. She is a research scientist working in the field of skeletal muscle. The primary focus of her research activities is on skeletal muscle regeneration. Dr. Gaina has been involved in several research projects funded by regional, national, and international public agencies. She is an author and/or co-author of over twenty scientific papers and conference abstracts, as well as three book chapters.

Contents

Preface

Molecular diagnostics has rapidly evolved from a specialized laboratory tool into a cornerstone of modern medicine. Advances in technology, bioinformatics, and molecular biology now allow us to detect and characterize diseases with unprecedented precision, shaping the future of personalized healthcare.

This book provides an overview of current molecular diagnostic technologies and their clinical applications. It highlights the evolution from conventional PCR to advanced methods such as quantitative PCR (qPCR), digital PCR (dPCR), and next-generation sequencing (NGS), each offering increasing sensitivity, specificity, and quantification capabilities. Key concepts such as liquid biopsy, cell-free nucleic acids, and non-invasive diagnostics are also discussed, along with their relevance in fields like oncology, prenatal medicine, and infectious disease.

We hope this work will serve as both a practical reference and a source of inspiration for professionals, researchers, and students dedicated to advancing diagnostic science.

We extend our sincere gratitude to our Publishing Process Manager, Maja Bozicevic, whose guidance, expertise, and commitment have been invaluable in bringing this book to completion.

Gisela Gaina
"Victor Babeș" National Institute of Pathology,
"Carol Davila" University of Medicine and Pharmacy,
Bucharest, Romania

Chapter 1

Introductory Chapter: Molecular Diagnostics in the Era of Precision Medicine

Gisela Gaina

1. Introduction

Genetic testing is an essential aspect of personalized medicine, allowing the identification and investigation of several biomarkers helpful to disease diagnosis, prognosis, and treatment response.

Over the past decade, substantial progress in molecular diagnostic technologies has profoundly influenced clinical practice by enhancing our understanding of the genetic and molecular pathways that underpin a broad spectrum of human diseases.

This rapidly evolving field focuses primarily on the detection and quantification of nucleic acids (DNA and RNA), offering high analytical sensitivity and specificity for early and precise disease characterization. A wide range of molecular techniques has evolved, building upon the foundational discovery by Kary Mullis, which introduced the polymerase chain reaction (PCR) and marked the beginning of modern molecular diagnostics [1]. Subsequent decades have witnessed significant advancements in these technologies, ultimately enabling faster diagnostic workflows and a deeper understanding of various pathological conditions.

In the years that followed, significant technical progress resulted in accelerated and more precise tests, alongside an enhanced understanding of diverse disease causes. These advancements have resulted in the emergence of highly sensitive and high-throughput techniques such as real-time PCR (qPCR), digital PCR, and next-generation sequencing (NGS) [2], which are currently essential instruments in both clinical and research settings.

The clinical applications of molecular diagnostic techniques have expanded rapidly, particularly in fields such as oncology, infectious diseases, and inherited genetic disorders. In oncology, for instance, molecular profiling of tumors enables the identification of specific gene mutations, translocations, or expression patterns that guide targeted therapies and prognostic assessments. In infectious disease diagnostics, real-time PCR and NGS enable quick and accurate detection of pathogens, including emerging or drug-resistant strains [3]. Furthermore, in the context of hereditary conditions, molecular analysis allows for early diagnosis, carrier screening, and prenatal testing, contributing to more informed clinical decision-making and personalized patient care [4].

Despite their transformative potential, molecular diagnostic techniques face several limitations that hinder widespread implementation in routine clinical practice. High costs associated with equipment, reagents, and data analysis platforms can limit access, particularly in low-resource settings. Additionally, the complexity of result interpretation—especially in next-generation sequencing—requires advanced bioinformatics support and specialized clinical expertise. Variability in regulatory frameworks, standardization protocols, and data quality control further complicates the integration of molecular diagnostics into healthcare systems. Ensuring equitable access and clinical utility remains a central challenge moving forward.

This chapter provides a concise overview of the current state of molecular diagnostic technology, including its advantages and disadvantages, practical applications, and associated costs. In particular, it explores the principles, strengths, and limitations of key molecular approaches—such as quantitative real-time PCR, droplet digital PCR, next-generation sequencing, and liquid biopsy—and their integration into clinical decision-making. Special attention is given to how these technologies have reshaped diagnostics in various diseases. By reviewing both established techniques and emerging innovations, this chapter aims to offer a comprehensive understanding of molecular diagnostics as a cornerstone of modern personalized medicine.

2. Current molecular diagnostic approaches

Human diseases encompass a wide and heterogeneous range of pathological phenotypes, each shaped by complex and often multifactorial pathogenic mechanisms. However, clinical classification systems commonly group disorders based on shared signs, symptoms, or histopathological features; the molecular underpinnings of these conditions may differ significantly across individuals or subtypes [5]. In many instances, distinct and seemingly unrelated biological pathways can give rise to similar clinical manifestations, such as inflammation, fibrosis, or cell death. This phenomenon illustrates the molecular heterogeneity that underlies uniform disease phenotypes. Furthermore, a single clinical entity may have multiple molecular subtypes, each characterized by unique genetic, transcriptomic, or epigenetic signatures [5]. Recognizing this diversity is essential for accurate diagnosis, effective treatment selection, and the advancement of personalized medicine, as it emphasizes the limitations of phenotype-based classification alone and highlights the need for molecular stratification of patients.

This molecular and clinical heterogeneity presents significant challenges for conventional diagnostic methods, which often rely solely on phenotypic manifestations or histological evaluation. As such, there is a growing need for diagnostic strategies that go beyond morphological descriptors and capture the underlying molecular signatures that determine disease onset and progression. By uncovering specific genetic, transcriptomic, or epigenetic alterations, molecular diagnostics enable a more nuanced and biologically informed classification of diseases, enabling earlier detection, improved prognostic assessment, and personalized therapeutic interventions [6].

Molecular diagnostics provides a robust framework for addressing the complexity of heterogeneous disease mechanisms by enabling the accurate identification of disease-specific molecular alterations. These approaches rely on detecting and quantifying nucleic acid sequences—DNA or RNA—with high specificity and sensitivity, thus offering a deeper understanding of disease classification and progression [7]. Among these tools, quantitative polymerase chain reaction (qPCR) remains a cornerstone method due to its speed, cost-effectiveness, and quantitative accuracy. More recently, digital PCR (dPCR) and droplet digital PCR (ddPCR) have enhanced the precision of nucleic acid quantification, especially in detecting low-abundance targets or mutations in complex or degraded samples. In parallel, modern diagnostics increasingly incorporate next-generation sequencing (NGS), microarray-based platforms, and liquid biopsy technologies, enabling genome-wide profiling, transcriptomic analysis, and the detection of molecular markers from non-invasive samples. These techniques have significantly expanded the clinical utility of molecular diagnostics, offering early detection, patient stratification, and real-time monitoring of treatment response. The following sections provide an overview of these technologies, their analytical principles, and their clinical applications across various disease contexts.

2.1 Polymerase chain reaction and its diagnostic utility

Since its introduction by Kary Mullis in the 1980s [1], the polymerase chain reaction (PCR) has become one of the most widely used and influential techniques in molecular biology and clinical diagnostics. PCR enables the exponential amplification of specific DNA sequences, allowing for the detection of nucleic acids with high specificity and sensitivity. PCR is widely used for detecting genetic mutations, identifying pathogens, genotyping, and analyzing inherited disorders. In clinical settings, PCR facilitates early diagnosis of infectious diseases, prenatal genetic screening, and confirmation of somatic mutations in cancer [8]. The technique's adaptability, speed, and relative cost-effectiveness have made it indispensable in both research and diagnostic settings. The technique's versatility and simplicity have led to numerous variations, including reverse transcription PCR (RT-PCR) for RNA analysis and quantitative PCR (qPCR) for real-time quantification of nucleic acids, further expanding its diagnostic utility.

Despite the emergence of high-throughput technologies, PCR continues to be a first-line diagnostic tool. Its enduring relevance underscores its critical role in the era of precision medicine and molecularly guided clinical decision-making. However, conventional PCR is primarily a qualitative method, providing presence-or-absence information without offering precise quantification. It also requires post-amplification steps such as gel electrophoresis, which increase contamination risk and processing time. These limitations have driven the development of more advanced amplification technologies, such as *quantitative real-time PCR (qPCR)* and *digital PCR (dPCR)*, which allow for more accurate, real-time quantification of nucleic acids.

2.2 Real-time PCR and quantitative PCR (qPCR)

Real-time PCR, and quantitative PCR (qPCR) variant, is a molecular technique that enables the detection and quantification of nucleic acids during the exponential phase of amplification. In contrast to conventional endpoint PCR, which detects amplicons only after the completion of all cycles, real-time PCR monitors the accumulation of target DNA in real time by measuring fluorescence emitted by intercalating dyes (e.g., SYBR Green) or sequence-specific probes (e.g., TaqMan). The intensity of the fluorescence signal directly correlates with the amount of nucleic acid present, allowing for either relative or absolute quantification, depending on assay design.

qPCR has become a cornerstone of molecular diagnostics, valued for its high sensitivity, specificity, and rapid turnaround time. Its ability to perform amplification and quantification in a closed-tube system minimizes contamination risk and makes it compatible with high-throughput diagnostic workflows. Clinically, qPCR is routinely employed in various disease testing such as HIV [9], SARS-CoV-2 [10], detection of somatic mutations e.g., BCR-AB gene expression profiling [11], and quantification of circulating microRNAs [12] or cell-free nucleic acids, [13].

Despite its versatility and broad adoption, qPCR presents several limitations. These include reduced accuracy at very low target concentrations, difficulties in detecting small fold-changes, and susceptibility to PCR inhibitors or sample variability. Additionally, the need for normalization against reference genes and the use of standard curves introduces variability in quantification. To overcome these challenges, *digital PCR (dPCR)* has emerged as a next-generation method offering absolute quantification without the need for reference standards or calibration curves. The following section will explore the principles and clinical relevance of this emerging technology.

2.3 Digital PCR (dPCR) and its droplet-based variant

Digital PCR (dPCR) represents a significant advancement in nucleic acid quantification, enabling absolute measurement of DNA or RNA molecules without the need for standard curves [14]. Unlike traditional qPCR, which provides relative quantification based on amplification kinetics, dPCR works by partitioning the sample into thousands or even millions of individual reactions, such that each partition contains either zero or one (or a few) target molecules. Following PCR amplification, partitions are scored as positive or negative, and the number of target molecules is calculated using Poisson statistics. Among the various dPCR platforms, droplet digital PCR (ddPCR) is the most widely adopted. In ddPCR, the sample is emulsified into nanoliter-sized droplets, each serving as an independent microreactor [15]. This technique provides high sensitivity, precision, and tolerance to PCR inhibitors, making it particularly valuable for applications such as rare mutation detection, quantification of low-abundance transcripts, microRNA profiling, and monitoring of minimal residual disease.

Numerous studies have highlighted the advantages of droplet digital PCR (ddPCR) in clinical and research settings, particularly in applications where sensitivity and absolute quantification are critical [14]. For instance, ddPCR has been successfully used to quantify circulating tumor DNA (ctDNA) in oncology, allowing detection of rare mutations such as *EGFR* T790M in non-small cell lung cancer patients, even at allele frequencies below 0.1% [16]. In virology, ddPCR has demonstrated superior accuracy in monitoring viral load in HIV and SARS-CoV-2, especially when conventional qPCR methods yielded inconclusive results due to low copy numbers [17]. In neurodegenerative research, ddPCR has been employed to measure microRNA expression levels in cerebrospinal fluid and brain tissue, providing reproducible data despite the presence of inhibitors common in complex biological matrices [18]. These findings consistently support ddPCR as a highly sensitive and reproducible method, with a strong potential to complement or even replace traditional qPCR in specific diagnostic and monitoring applications.

Droplet digital PCR (ddPCR) has also emerged as a powerful tool for quantifying exon skipping efficiency in RNA-based therapeutic strategies, particularly in the context of neuromuscular disorders such as Duchenne muscular dystrophy (DMD). Exon skipping aims to restore the reading frame of defective mRNAs by using antisense oligonucleotides (AONs) to exclude specific exons during splicing. ddPCR allows for precise quantification of both skipped and non-skipped transcript isoforms, even when present at low levels [19], by using isoform-specific primer-probe sets. Compared to conventional RT-qPCR, ddPCR provides absolute counts of target molecules, increased reproducibility, and better sensitivity in detecting subtle changes in splicing patterns. Several studies have validated ddPCR as a reliable method for measuring exon skipping efficiency in preclinical and clinical settings, supporting its use in monitoring therapeutic response and optimizing dosing regimens for exon-skipping agents [20, 21].

While digital PCR has significantly advanced the precision of nucleic acid quantification, its utility remains limited to known sequences and predefined targets. To explore broader genetic landscapes, detect novel variants, or analyze complex transcriptomes, more comprehensive approaches are required [22]. To overcome these limitations and to enable the discovery of novel variants, structural rearrangements, and global expression changes, high-throughput sequencing technologies—such as next-generation sequencing (NGS)—have become essential tools in modern molecular diagnostics.

2.4 Sequencing

Sequencing is a fundamental technique in molecular biology that enables the determination of the precise order of nucleotides in DNA or RNA molecules [23]. Over time, sequencing technologies have evolved from first-generation methods such as Sanger sequencing to high-throughput approaches like next-generation sequencing (NGS) and, more recently, third-generation platforms, including nanopore and single-molecule real-time (SMRT) sequencing [24]. While Sanger sequencing remains valuable for small-scale, high-accuracy applications [25], NGS allows for parallel sequencing of millions of fragments, enabling genome-wide analyses. Third-generation sequencing adds the advantage of long-read capabilities, which is useful in structural variant detection and complex genome assembly [26]. Together, these technologies have revolutionized diagnostics, personalized medicine, and biomedical research by enabling comprehensive and detailed insights into genetic and epigenetic landscapes.

A landmark study published in *Nature Communications* [27] highlighted the clinical value of third-generation long-read sequencing (LRS) in genetic diagnostics. Researchers implemented an innovative analytical workflow that combined filters for single nucleotide variants (SNVs), structural variations, and genome-wide epigenetic patterns. In a positive control cohort (n = 76), the method successfully identified all known pathogenic variants, including SNVs, rearrangements, and methylation changes. Among 51 patients who had previously received no diagnosis through conventional short-read methods, LRS provided additional diagnostic insights in 10% of cases, notably uncovering epigenetic signatures relevant to spinal muscular atrophy. This study underscores the potential of LRS as a feasible "all-in-one" approach for clinical genetic diagnostics and rare disease variant discovery.

Despite their transformative capabilities, sequencing technologies face several challenges, including high costs, data interpretation complexity, storage burden, and the need for sophisticated bioinformatics pipelines. Additionally, incidental findings or variants of uncertain significance (VUS) raise ethical and clinical interpretation issues that require cautious management in diagnostic workflows [28].

2.5 Liquid biopsy/cell-free DNA (cfDNA) assay/ctDNA/diagnostic prenatal

Liquid biopsy is a minimally invasive diagnostic approach that enables the detection and analysis of molecular biomarkers—such as circulating tumor DNA (ctDNA), cell-free RNA, exosomes, and circulating tumor cells (CTCs)—from body fluids, most commonly blood [29]. Unlike traditional tissue biopsies, which require invasive sampling of solid tumors, liquid biopsies offer a real-time snapshot of systemic disease, allowing for longitudinal monitoring of tumor evolution, treatment response, and minimal residual disease [30]. This technique has proven especially valuable in oncology [31], where it supports early cancer detection, identification of actionable mutations, and detection of resistance mechanisms [31]. Beyond cancer, liquid biopsy is increasingly explored in areas such as prenatal diagnostics, organ transplantation, and neurodegenerative disease, highlighting its broad potential in personalized medicine and noninvasive disease management [32, 33].

Cell-free DNA (cfDNA) analysis has revolutionized non-invasive prenatal testing (NIPT) by enabling early detection of fetal genetic abnormalities from maternal blood samples [34]. Originating primarily from placental trophoblasts, fetal cfDNA represents a small fraction of the total circulating DNA in maternal plasma, typically as low as 5–15% in early pregnancy [35]. To accurately detect chromosomal aneuploidies such as trisomy 21, 18, and 13—or even single-gene disorders—analytical techniques must achieve exceptional sensitivity and specificity [36]. *Droplet digital PCR (ddPCR)* has proven particularly useful in this context due to its ability to perform absolute quantification of rare fetal alleles within a high maternal DNA background. Unlike conventional qPCR, ddPCR partitions the sample into thousands of nanoliter droplets, improving resolution and detection limits. Studies have shown that ddPCR-based assays can distinguish subtle allelic imbalances, detect paternal mutations inherited by the fetus, and even quantify fetal fraction, making it a valuable complement or alternative to next-generation sequencing in targeted prenatal applications [37].

As liquid biopsy technologies continue to evolve, their integration into routine clinical workflows offers the promise of earlier diagnosis [38], more precise risk stratification [39], and dynamic monitoring of disease. While challenges remain—such as standardization, cost-effectiveness, and data interpretation—ongoing advances in digital PCR, sequencing, and bioinformatics are rapidly addressing these barriers. The growing clinical utility of liquid biopsy underscores its central role in the future of noninvasive molecular diagnostics. Moreover, emerging multi-analyte approaches that combine cfDNA, cfRNA, and protein biomarkers from the same sample are paving the way for more comprehensive molecular profiling from a single liquid biopsy.

3. Technical considerations in molecular diagnostics

The accuracy and reproducibility of molecular diagnostic assays are highly dependent on multiple technical factors. One critical element is the quality and quantity of nucleic acids extracted from clinical specimens [40]. Low input material, degraded samples, or contamination with host DNA or RNases can significantly impact assay sensitivity and reliability—particularly in applications like liquid biopsy, where analytes, such as cfDNA and microRNAs, are present at low concentrations [41].

Pre-analytical variables, including sample type, collection method, transport conditions, and processing time, can introduce variability that affects downstream analyses. For instance, improper handling of blood samples may lead to leukocyte lysis, releasing genomic DNA that dilutes or masks cell-free DNA signals. Similarly, RNA-based assays are particularly sensitive to degradation and require stringent stabilization protocols [42].

In amplification-based methods, PCR inhibitors (e.g., heme, bile salts, EDTA) may interfere with enzyme activity and yield false negatives or quantification bias. The implementation of internal controls, proper normalization strategies, and rigorous quality control measures is essential to mitigate these issues. Standardization of sample processing workflows and validation of analytical performance across laboratories remain key for reliable clinical implementation [43, 44].

The clinical implementation of molecular diagnostic tests must comply with international quality and regulatory standards to ensure analytical validity, reproducibility, and clinical relevance. For quantitative PCR (qPCR), adherence to the *MIQE guidelines* (*Minimum Information for Publication of Quantitative Real-Time PCR Experiments*) [45] is strongly recommended to ensure experimental transparency, reproducibility, and accurate data interpretation.

Clinical laboratories offering molecular testing must follow quality assurance frameworks **ISO 15189** [46], which establish criteria for test validation, personnel qualifications, and quality control procedures.

For genomic tests using next-generation sequencing (NGS), variant interpretation must follow professional guidelines such as those provided by the *American College of Medical Genetics and Genomics (ACMG)*, [47] which define classification criteria for pathogenicity and clinical significance. Integration of these standards is essential for ensuring reliable molecular results that inform patient care.

4. Challenges and future directions

While molecular diagnostics have transformed clinical practice, several challenges remain. High costs, particularly for NGS and dPCR platforms, limit accessibility in low-resource settings. Additionally, the interpretation of complex data—such as variants of uncertain significance or incidental findings—requires specialized bioinformatics support and clinical expertise. The lack of assay standardization and inter-laboratory reproducibility further complicates broad clinical adoption.

Despite these limitations, the field is moving toward multi-omic integration and AI-driven analysis, aiming to provide more holistic and predictive insights into disease. Portable and point-of-care molecular tools, including handheld sequencers and simplified PCR devices, are also emerging, with potential to democratize diagnostics globally. As technologies mature and become more affordable, molecular diagnostics are expected to become central to personalized, preventative, and precision medicine.

5. Conclusions

Molecular diagnostics have redefined the landscape of modern medicine by enabling precise, rapid, and minimally invasive detection of genetic and molecular alterations. From PCR-based methods to next-generation sequencing and liquid biopsy, these technologies support early diagnosis, treatment personalization, and real-time disease monitoring across a wide range of clinical domains. While challenges related to cost, data interpretation, and standardization remain, ongoing innovations—particularly in digital PCR, long-read sequencing, and AI-assisted analytics—are rapidly addressing these barriers. As molecular diagnostics continue to evolve, they are poised to play a central role in delivering predictive, personalized, and preventive healthcare.

Acknowledgements

The author would like to thank National Program 1 N/2023/PN 23.16.01.02 for supporting this project.

Conflict of interest

The authors declare no conflict of interest.

Abbreviations

PCR:	polymerase chain reaction
RT-PCR:	reverse transcription polymerase chain reaction
qPCR:	quantitative real-time PCR
dPCR:	digital PCR
ddPCR:	droplet digital PCR
NGS:	next-generation sequencing
SMRT:	single-molecule real-time (sequencing)
LRS:	long-read sequencing
cfDNA:	cell-free DNA
ctDNA:	circulating tumor DNA
CTCs:	circulating tumor cells
NIPT:	non-invasive prenatal testing
AONs:	antisense oligonucleotides
MIQE:	minimum information for publication of quantitative real-time PCR experiments
ISO 15189:	international organization for standardization, medical laboratories-requirements for quality and competence
ACMG:	American college of medical genetics and genomics
VUS:	variants of uncertain significance
AI:	artificial intelligence

Author details

Gisela Gaina[1,2]

1 “Victor Babeş” National Institute of Pathology, Bucharest, Romania

2 “Carol Davila” University of Medicine and Pharmacy, Bucharest, Romania

*Address all correspondence to: gisela.gaina@ivb.ro

References

[1] Mullis KB, Faloona FA. Specific synthesis of DNA in vitro via the polymerase catalyzed reaction. Methods Enzymol. 1987;**155**:335-350

[2] Metzker ML. Sequencing technologies — The next generation. Nature Reviews. Genetics [Internet]. 2010;**11**(1):31-46. Available from: https://www.nature.com/articles/nrg2626

[3] Farhat J, Alzyoud L, AlWahsh M, Acharjee A, Al-Omari B. Advancing precision medicine: The role of genetic testing and sequencing technologies in identifying biological markers for rare cancers. Cancer Medicine. Apr 2025;**14**(8):e70853. DOI: 10.1002/cam4.70853

[4] Pillai RK, Jayasree K. Rare cancers. The Indian Journal of Medical Research. 2017;**145**(1):17-27. Available from: https://ijmr.org.in/rare-cancers-challenges-issues/

[5] Loscalzo J, Kohane I, Barabasi AL. Human disease classification in the postgenomic era: A complex systems approach to human pathobiology. Molecular Systems Biology. 2007;**3**:124. DOI: 10.1038/msb4100163

[6] Malhotra GK, Zhao X, Band H, Band V. Histological, molecular and functional subtypes of breast cancers. Cancer Biology & Therapy [Internet]. 2010;**10**(10):955-960. DOI: 10.4161/cbt.10.10.13879

[7] Khodakov D, Wang C, Zhang DY. Diagnostics based on nucleic acid sequence variant profiling: PCR, hybridization, and NGS approaches. Advanced Drug Delivery Reviews [Internet]. 2016;**105**:3-19. Available from: https://linkinghub.elsevier.com/retrieve/pii/S0169409X16301041

[8] Liu Q, Jin X, Cheng J, Zhou H, Zhang Y, Dai Y. Advances in the application of molecular diagnostic techniques for the detection of infectious disease pathogens (review). Molecular Medicine Reports [Internet]. 2023;**27**(5):104. Available from: http://www.spandidos-publications.com/10.3892/mmr.2023.12991

[9] Mellors JW, Kingsley LA, Rinaldo CR, Todd JA, Hoo BS, Kokka RP, et al. Quantitation of HIV-1 RNA in plasma predicts outcome after seroconversion. Annals of Internal Medicine [Internet]. 1995;**122**(8):573-579. DOI: 10.7326/0003-4819-122-8-199504150-00003

[10] Dutta D, Naiyer S, Mansuri S, Soni N, Singh V, Bhat KH, et al. COVID-19 diagnosis: A comprehensive review of the RT-qPCR method for detection of SARS-CoV-2. Diagnostics [Internet]. 2022;**12**(6):1503. Available from: https://www.mdpi.com/2075-4418/12/6/1503

[11] Alikian M, Gale RP, Apperley JF, Foroni L. Molecular techniques for the personalised management of patients with chronic myeloid leukaemia. Biomolecular Detection and Quantification [Internet]. 2017;**11**:4-20. Available from: https://linkinghub.elsevier.com/retrieve/pii/S2214753517300013

[12] Metcalf GAD. MicroRNAs: Circulating biomarkers for the early detection of imperceptible cancers via biosensor and machine-learning advances. Oncogene [Internet]. 2024;**43**(28):2135-2142. Available from: https://www.nature.com/articles/s41388-024-03076-3

[13] Sultana GNN, Akter F, Israfil SMH, Ray UC, Jahan RA, Ali MS, et al. Quantitative analysis of serum cell-free DNA as a predictive and prognostic marker in breast cancer patients. Frontiers in Oncology. 22 Jun 2023;**13**:1171412. DOI: 10.3389/fonc.2023.1171412

[14] Mirabile A, Sangiorgio G, Bonacci PG, Bivona D, Nicitra E, Bonomo C, et al. Advancing pathogen identification: The role of digital PCR in enhancing diagnostic power in different settings. Diagnostics [Internet]. 2024;**14**(15):1598. Available from: https://www.mdpi.com/2075-4418/14/15/1598

[15] Kojabad AA, Farzanehpour M, Galeh HEG, Dorostkar R, Jafarpour A, Bolandian M, et al. Droplet digital PCR of viral DNA/RNA, current progress, challenges, and future perspectives. Journal of Medical Virology [Internet]. 2021;**93**(7):4182-4197. DOI: 10.1002/jmv.26846

[16] Durgut S, Salihefendić L, Pećar D, Čeko I, Mulahuseinović N, Izmirlija M, et al. Droplet digital PCR as a molecular tool for the detection of the EGFR T790M mutation in NSCLC patients with the EGFR activating mutations. Balkan Journal of Medical Genetics : BJMG [Internet]. 2023;**26**(2):21-26. DOI: 10.2478/bjmg-2023-0020

[17] Vasudevan HN, Xu P, Servellita V, Miller S, Liu L, Gopez A, et al. Digital droplet PCR accurately quantifies SARS-CoV-2 viral load from crude lysate without nucleic acid purification. Scientific Reports [Internet]. 2021;**11**(1):780. Available from: https://www.nature.com/articles/s41598-020-80715-1

[18] Trypsteen W, Kiselinova M, Vandekerckhove L, De Spiegelaere W. Diagnostic utility of droplet digital PCR for HIV reservoir quantification. Journal of Virus Eradication [Internet]. 2016;**2**(3):162-169. Available from: https://linkinghub.elsevier.com/retrieve/pii/S205566402030460X

[19] Verheul RC, Van Deutekom JCT, Datson NA. Digital droplet PCR for the absolute quantification of exon skipping induced by antisense oligonucleotides in (pre-)clinical development for duchenne muscular dystrophy. PLoS One. 2016;**11**(9):1-18

[20] Hiller M, Falzarano MS, Garcia-Jimenez I, Sardone V, Verheul RC, Popplewell L, et al. A multicenter comparison of quantification methods for antisense oligonucleotide-induced DMD exon 51 skipping in Duchenne muscular dystrophy cell cultures. PLoS One [Internet]. 2018;**13**(10):e0204485. Available from: http://www.ncbi.nlm.nih.gov/pubmed/30278058

[21] Spitali P, Heemskerk H, Vossen RH, Ferlini A, den Dunnen JT, 't Hoen PA, et al. Accurate quantification of dystrophin mRNA and exon skipping levels in Duchenne muscular dystrophy. Laboratory Investigation. 2010;**90**(September):1396-1402

[22] Coccaro N, Tota G, Anelli L, Zagaria A, Specchia G, Albano F. Digital PCR: A Reliable Tool for Analyzing and Monitoring Hematologic Malignancies. International Journal of Molecular Sciences. 29 Apr 2020;**21**(9):3141. DOI: 10.3390/ijms21093141

[23] Heather JM, Chain B. The sequence of sequencers: The history of sequencing DNA. Genomics [Internet]. 2016;**107**(1):1-8. Available from: https://linkinghub.elsevier.com/retrieve/pii/S0888754315300410

[24] Slatko BE, Gardner AF, Ausubel FM. Overview of next-generation sequencing

technologies. Current Protocols in Molecular Biology. Apr 2018;**122**(1):e59. DOI: 10.1002/cpmb.59

[25] Sanger F, Coulson AR. A rapid method for determining sequences in DNA by primed synthesis with DNA polymerase. Journal of Molecular Biology [Internet]. 1975;**94**(3):441-448. Available from: https://linkinghub.elsevier.com/retrieve/pii/0022283675902132

[26] Satam H, Joshi K, Mangrolia U, Waghoo S, Zaidi G, Rawool S, et al. Next-generation sequencing technology: Current trends and advancements. Biology (Basel) [Internet]. 2023;**12**(7):997. Available from: https://www.mdpi.com/2079-7737/12/7/997

[27] Sinha S, Rabea F, Ramaswamy S, Chekroun I, El Naofal M, Jain R, et al. Long read sequencing enhances pathogenic and novel variation discovery in patients with rare diseases. Nature Communications [Internet]. 2025;**16**(1):2500. Available from: https://www.nature.com/articles/s41467-025-57695-9

[28] Van den Veyver IB, Chandler N, Wilkins-Haug LE, Wapner RJ, Chitty LS. International Society for Prenatal Diagnosis Updated Position Statement on the use of genome-wide sequencing for prenatal diagnosis. Prenatal Diagnosis [Internet]. 2022;**42**(6):796-803. DOI: 10.1002/pd.6157

[29] Alix-Panabières C, Pantel K. Clinical applications of circulating tumor cells and circulating tumor DNA as liquid biopsy. Cancer Discovery [Internet]. 2016;**6**(5):479-491. Available from: https://aacrjournals.org/cancerdiscovery/article/6/5/479/5481/Clinical-Applications-of-Circulating-Tumor-Cells

[30] Wan JCM, Massie C, Garcia-Corbacho J, Mouliere F, Brenton JD, Caldas C, et al. Liquid biopsies come of age: Towards implementation of circulating tumour DNA. Nature Reviews. Cancer [Internet]. 2017;**17**(4):223-238. Available from: https://www.nature.com/articles/nrc.2017.7

[31] Siravegna G, Marsoni S, Siena S, Bardelli A. Integrating liquid biopsies into the management of cancer. Nature Reviews. Clinical Oncology [Internet]. 2017;**14**(9):531-548. Available from: https://www.nature.com/articles/nrclinonc.2017.14

[32] Lo YMD, Han DSC, Jiang P, Chiu RWK. Epigenetics, fragmentomics, and topology of cell-free DNA in liquid biopsies. Science. 9 Apr 2021;**372**(6538):eaaw3616. DOI: 10.1126/science.aaw3616

[33] Sun K, Jiang P, Chan KC, Wong J, Cheng YK, Liang RH, et al. Plasma DNA tissue mapping by genome-wide methylation sequencing for noninvasive prenatal, cancer, and transplantation assessments. Proceedings of the National Academy of Sciences USA. 6 Oct 2015;**112**(40):E5503-12. DOI: 10.1073/pnas.1508736112. Epub 2015 Sep 21

[34] Bianchi DW, Parker RL, Wentworth J, Madankumar R, Saffer C, Das AF, et al. DNA sequencing versus standard prenatal aneuploidy screening. The New England Journal of Medicine [Internet]. 2014;**370**(9):799-808. DOI: 10.1056/NEJMoa1311037

[35] Silver R, Myatt L, Hauth J, Leveno K, Peaceman A, Ramin S, et al. Cell-free Total and Fetal DNA in first trimester maternal serum and subsequent development of preeclampsia. American Journal of Perinatology [Internet]. 2016;**34**(02):191-198. DOI: 10.1055/s-0035-1570383

[36] Guo Y, Charoenkwan P, Traisrisilp K, Piyamongkol W, Tongprasert F. Application

of digital polymerase Chain reaction (dPCR) in non-invasive prenatal testing (NIPT). Biomolecules [Internet]. 2025;**15**(3):360. Available from: https://www.mdpi.com/2218-273X/15/3/360

[37] D'Aversa E, Breveglieri G, Pellegatti P, Guerra G, Gambari R, Borgatti M. Non-invasive fetal sex diagnosis in plasma of early weeks pregnants using droplet digital PCR. Molecular Medicine [Internet]. 2018;**24**(1):14. DOI: 10.1186/s10020-018-0016-7

[38] Chen Z, Li C, Zhou Y, Yao Y, Liu J, Wu M, et al. Liquid biopsies for cancer: From bench to clinic. MedComm (2020). 23 Jul 2023;**4**(4):e329. DOI: 10.1002/mco2.329

[39] Ganig N, Baenke F, Thepkaysone M-L, Lin K, Rao VS, Wong FC, et al. Proteomic analyses of fibroblast- and serum-derived exosomes identify QSOX1 as a marker for non-invasive detection of colorectal cancer. Cancers (Basel) [Internet]. 2021;**13**(6):1351. Available from: https://www.mdpi.com/2072-6694/13/6/1351

[40] Anvari M, Gharib A, Abolhasani M, Azari-Yaam A, Gharalari F, Safavi M, et al. Pre-analytical practices in the molecular diagnostic tests, a concise review. Iranian Journal of Pathology [Internet]. 2021;**16**(1):1-19. Available from: http://ijp.iranpath.org/article_46859.html

[41] Li L, Sun Y. Circulating tumor DNA methylation detection as biomarker and its application in tumor liquid biopsy: Advances and challenges. MedComm (2020). 9 Nov 2024;**5**(11):e766. DOI: 10.1002/mco2.766

[42] Peng H, Pan M, Zhou Z, Chen C, Xing X, Cheng S, et al. The impact of preanalytical variables on the analysis of cell-free DNA from blood and urine samples. Frontiers in Cell and Development Biology. 9 May 2024;**12**:1385041. DOI: 10.3389/fcell.2024.1385041

[43] Sidstedt M, Rådström P, Hedman J. PCR inhibition in qPCR, dPCR and MPS—Mechanisms and solutions. Analytical and Bioanalytical Chemistry [Internet]. 2020;**412**(9):2009-2023. DOI: 10.1007/s00216-020-02490-2

[44] Buckwalter SP, Sloan LM, Cunningham SA, Espy MJ, Uhl JR, Jones MF, et al. Inhibition controls for qualitative real-time PCR assays: Are they necessary for all specimen matrices? Journal of Clinical Microbiology [Internet]. 2014;**52**(6):2139-2143. DOI: 10.1128/JCM.03389-13

[45] Bustin SA, Benes V, Garson JA, Hellemans J, Huggett J, Kubista M, et al. The MIQE guidelines: Minimum information for publication of quantitative real-time PCR experiments. Clinical Chemistry. 2009;**55**(4):611-622

[46] Schneider F, Maurer C, Friedberg RC. International Organization for Standardization (ISO) 15189. Annals of Laboratory Medicine [Internet]. 2017;**37**(5):365-370. DOI: 10.3343/alm.2017.37.5.365

[47] Richards S, Aziz N, Bale S, Bick D, Das S, Gastier-Foster J, et al. Standards and guidelines for the interpretation of sequence variants: A joint consensus recommendation of the American College of Medical Genetics and Genomics and the Association for Molecular Pathology. Genetics in Medicine [Internet]. 2015;**17**(5):405-424. Available from: https://linkinghub.elsevier.com/retrieve/pii/S1098360021030318

Chapter 2

Revolutionizing Dentistry with Molecular Diagnostics

Gopal Nath and Alka Shukla

Abstract

Molecular diagnostics plays a pivotal role in contemporary dentistry by leveraging advanced methodologies to detect and characterize genetic sequences, pathogenic microorganisms, and biomarkers within dental and oral tissues. It facilitates a deeper understanding of the etiological factors and pathological progression of various oromaxillofacial conditions, including periodontal diseases, oral carcinomas, and microbial infections. Techniques such as Polymerase Chain Reaction (PCR) and next-generation sequencing (NGS) enable the precise identification of specific pathogens, genetic mutations, and molecular risk factors at a granular level. These diagnostic approaches offer unparalleled sensitivity, specificity, and the potential for early detection, thereby enabling the formulation of personalized therapeutic strategies and enhancing clinical outcomes. This technological advancement holds significant promise for revolutionizing both preventive and interventional care within the field of dentistry. Ultimately, this innovation holds the potential to redefine the way dental professionals approach diagnosis, prevention, and treatment, leading to a more proactive and individualized model of care. This chapter will thoroughly explore the various facets of molecular diagnostics, highlighting their potential applications and transformative impact within the field of dentistry. It will cover the latest advancements, techniques, and the role of molecular tools in enhancing diagnostic accuracy and treatment outcomes.

Keywords: molecular diagnostics, oral biofilm, genetic disorders, polymerase chain reaction, genome sequencing

1. Introduction

Oral cavity pathologies, encompassing a wide range of conditions such as periodontal diseases, oral cancers, and infections, affect millions of individuals globally [1, 2]. These ailments lead to significant morbidity, impairing individuals' quality of life, and in severe cases, resulting in mortality. The global burden of oral diseases highlights their profound impact on public health, demanding comprehensive prevention and treatment strategies to mitigate their consequences. Among the notable advancements aimed at addressing this challenge, molecular diagnostics has emerged as a powerful tool, offering precise, early detection and improved management of oral health conditions.

IntechOpen

2. Overview of molecular diagnostics

Molecular diagnostics (MD) is a rapidly advancing field within clinical laboratory medicine that applies molecular biology techniques to detect and quantify nucleic acid sequences and protein-based biomarkers associated with disease. It plays a pivotal role in the diagnosis, prognosis, and therapeutic monitoring of a wide spectrum of conditions, including infectious diseases, genetic disorders, and malignancies. MD assays target molecular components such as genomic DNA, messenger RNA (mRNA), and proteins to uncover the underlying mechanisms of disease, enabling the identification of pathogenic variants, evaluation of disease progression, prediction of individual susceptibility, and assessment of treatment response. Analytical methods in MD include nucleic acid sequencing, epigenetic analysis (e.g., DNA methylation), transcriptomic profiling, proteomic analysis, and multiplex biomarker detection. The integration of these molecular indicators provides high-resolution insights into genotypic and phenotypic alterations, facilitating precise, personalized clinical decision-making [3].

In recent years, molecular diagnostics has transformed healthcare, extending its applications beyond general medicine into specialized fields such as dentistry. In dentistry, MD techniques are increasingly employed to identify oral pathogens, genetic predispositions, and systemic conditions with oral manifestations. By analyzing DNA, RNA, proteins, and other biomarkers, these diagnostics offer critical insights into the molecular etiology, pathophysiology, and progression of oral diseases. This has not only improved diagnostic accuracy and treatment outcomes but has also enhanced disease prevention strategies [4, 5]. This chapter will explore the growing role of molecular diagnostics in dental medicine, emphasizing its impact on patient care and its contribution to the advancement of oral healthcare.

3. Fundamentals of molecular techniques in dentistry

Molecular diagnostics is an advanced and highly sensitive field, founded on the three pillars of genomics, proteomics, and metabolomics (**Figure 1**) [6].

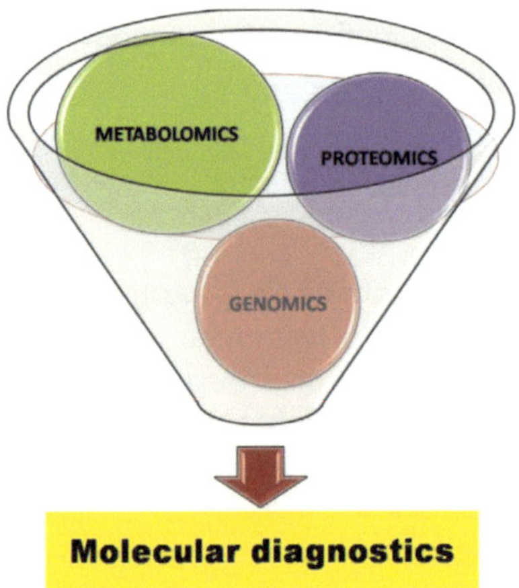

Figure 1.
Fundamentals of molecular diagnostics. Source: Author's original work (using Microsoft Office).

a. *Genomics*: It is the study of genes and their roles, encompassing the identification of an organism's genetic makeup and the exploration of gene functions through advanced biotechnological techniques. It has laid a solid groundwork for research in both human health and disease [7].

b. *Proteomics*: Proteomics is the analysis of extensive arrays of proteins within biological systems [8]. Various techniques for studying proteins include two-dimensional gel electrophoresis (2D-PAGE), liquid chromatography, mass spectrometry, and others [9].

c. *Metabolomics*: It is a systemic study that involves thorough examination and measurement of metabolites within a biological sample. In contrast to genomic and proteomic approaches, it focuses on quantifying molecules with diverse physical properties [10]. Metabolites are regarded as close indicators of disease, as their concentrations in biological samples are frequently closely linked to underlying pathogenic processes [11].

Dentistry can leverage the advantages of these three foundational pillars in the following ways: Genomic studies such as nucleic acid sequencing can detect bacterial genes responsible for virulence or genetic mutations associated with malignant tumors in the oral cavity, while proteomics facilitates the identification of infection-specific biomarkers, such as proteins, through techniques like enzyme-linked immunosorbent assay (ELISA). Metabolomics has emerged as a valuable tool for elucidating the body's response to diseases and is increasingly applied in the development of screening and diagnostic tools for cancer and other pathologies [12, 13].

The integration of these pillars offers a comprehensive approach to understanding oral health and disease. By combining these omics technologies, researchers and clinicians can obtain a broader and more detailed spectrum of molecular information, enabling more accurate diagnosis, personalized treatment planning, and improved prognostic evaluations in dentistry. This multiomics strategy enhances the ability to identify complex interactions among genes, proteins, and metabolic pathways, ultimately contributing to more effective and targeted interventions for oral diseases.

4. Various domains of molecular diagnostic applications in dentistry

Molecular diagnostics have profoundly advanced the medical field, including dentistry, facilitating more accurate, efficient, and individualized care. This technology offers a broad spectrum of applications in dentistry, providing innovative approaches for diagnosis, prevention, treatment, and research. **Figure 2** illustrates several key applications.

4.1 Investigations and diagnostics

In addition to conventional methods, advanced diagnostic techniques play a crucial role in establishing the diagnosis of oral diseases and disorders. Various molecular diagnostic techniques will be discussed in the upcoming sections. Below are the areas where molecular diagnostics can be applied to investigate and improve the quality of diagnosis.

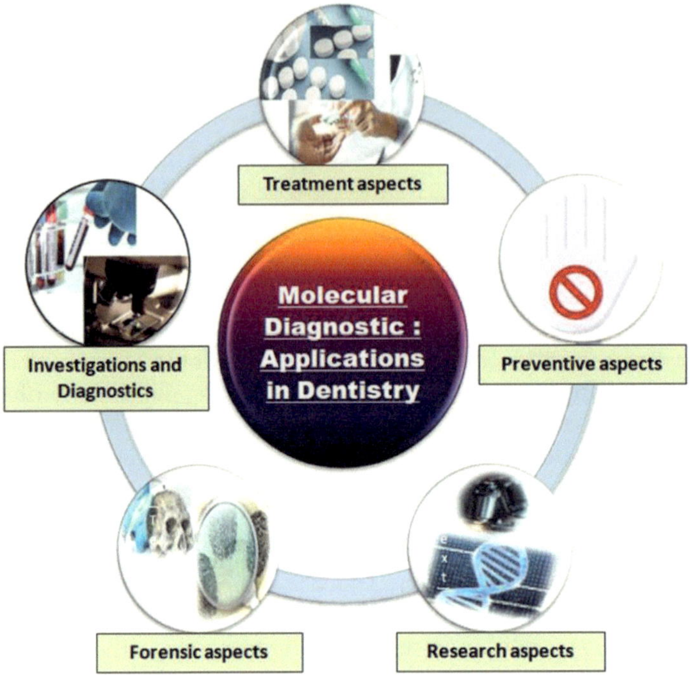

Figure 2.
Various dimensions of dentistry with potential applications of molecular diagnostics. Source: Author's original work (using Microsoft Office).

4.1.1 Detection of oral pathogens involved in oral disease

The oral cavity harbors a complex and diverse microbiota, encompassing bacteria, fungi, mycoplasma, protozoa, and potentially viral entities, with bacteria constituting the predominant microbial group. These microorganisms have the capacity to trigger a variety of infectious pathologies, as illustrated in **Figure 3** [14]. Certain oral diseases, including periodontitis, are attributed to a complex microbiota involving gram-positive and gram-negative bacteria [15, 16]. To ensure effective treatment, it is essential to identify the specific microbes involved. Further, molecular characterization of antibiotic-resistant strains aids in identifying unusual resistant strains and detecting new outbreak strains at an early stage [17]. Infection detection can be carried out in two ways: direct detection of oral pathogens, which involves two approaches—nucleic acid-based detection and protein/antigen-focused methods—and indirect diagnosis through the detection of the patient's immune response to the infection.

i Direct detection of oral pathogens

- The nucleic acid detection-centric approach: As illustrated in **Figure 4**, the nucleic acid-targeting methods involve fluorescence amplification techniques, such as polymerase chain reaction (PCR), quantitative or real-time PCR (qPCR), digital PCR (dPCR), DNA microarrays, fluorescence in situ hybridization (FISH), loop-mediated isothermal amplification (LAMP), and sequencing technologies like pyrosequencing, Illumina sequencing, and nanopore sequencing [18, 19].

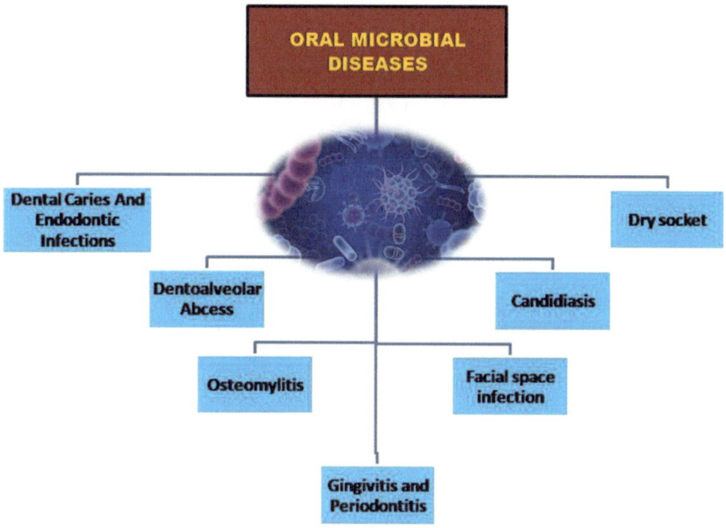

Figure 3.
Microbial infections *of the oral cavity. Source: Author's original work (using Microsoft Office).*

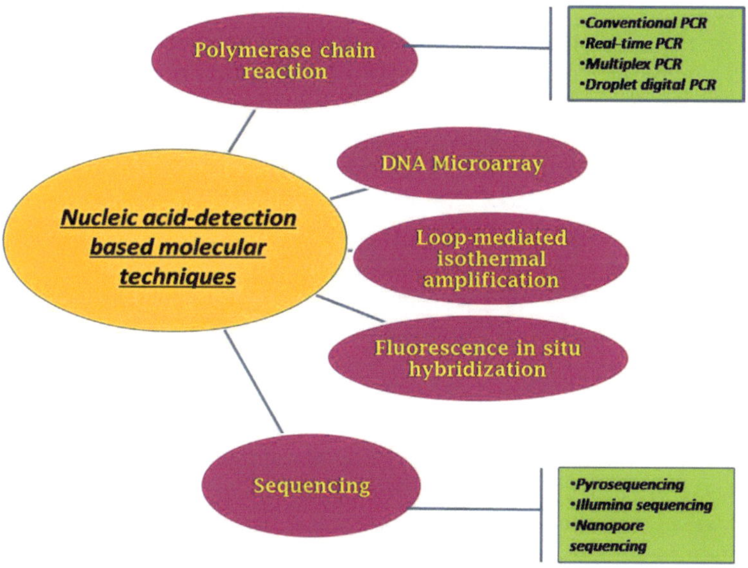

Figure 4.
Diverse molecular techniques for nucleic acid detection. Source: Author's original work (using Microsoft Office).

- The protein/antigen-focused approach involves traditional antibody-antigen interaction techniques, akin to immunological methods such as lateral flow tests (LFTs) and enzyme-linked immunosorbent assays (ELISA), immunofluorescence assays (IFA), and serum neutralization tests (SNTs). Additionally, by integrating fundamental molecular detection methods with metal and paper platforms, biosensor-based and paper-based devices have evolved into portable, on-site solutions [18].

ii Indirect diagnosis of infection

- The detection of pathogen-specific IgM is a commonly used method for confirming acute infection. Example: An available diagnostic kit uses an oral specimen collection device to gather HIV-1 antibodies from the cheek and gingiva [20].

4.1.2 Diagnosis of systemic diseases, disorders, and infections using oral samples

Saliva has been suggested as a diagnostic fluid also for systemic diseases such as diabetes, autoimmune disorders, viral and bacterial infections, as well as cardiovascular diseases. PCR also helps in diagnosing a variety of systemic viral infections such as SARS-CoV-2, influenza, and mumps, often utilizing oral or oropharyngeal swabs [21, 22].

4.1.3 Detection of biomarkers in saliva

Saliva is increasingly recognized as a valuable source of biological markers, containing alterations in biochemicals, DNA, RNA, proteins, and microbiota composition. The levels of macrophage inflammatory protein-1α, matrix metalloproteinase-8, interleukin-1β (IL-1β), IL-6, prostaglandin E2, and tumor necrosis factor-α (TNF-α) in saliva are closely associated with gingivitis and periodontitis, showing strong potential as biomarkers for diagnosing these periodontal diseases [23]. Matrix metalloproteinase-8 (MMP-8) is a crucial biomarker for periodontitis and peri-implantitis in oral fluids; thus, it can be a valuable biological tool for predicting these conditions [24–26]. Rich in bioactive metabolites, it has emerged as a promising, noninvasive, and cost-effective biomarker for disease detection, thereby assisting in the diagnosis of various systemic conditions [27, 28]. For instance, Sjögren's syndrome, an autoimmune systemic disorder, is linked to significant changes in the proteome and transcriptome, including marked alterations in the levels of IL-4, IL-5, and cytokine clusters [29]. Salivary components such as C-erbB2, CA 15-3, Cathepsin D, sialic acid, P53, EGF, VEGF, and CEA show potential as salivary biomarkers, which could be highly beneficial for detecting breast cancer and tracking patient progress after therapy [30].

4.1.4 Early detection of malignancy in oral tissue

Oropharyngeal carcinoma is classified among the most aggressive malignancies, with a survival rate of approximately 50%. Despite the oral cavity being readily accessible for visual examination, oral cancers are often diagnosed at later stages, with up to 50% remaining undetected until the disease has progressed significantly [31, 32]. It is widely recognized that tumors develop through a multistep process driven by the accumulation of genetic mutations [33]. The analysis of the genome, transcripts, and proteome holds significant promise in offering insights into cellular events that occur before clinically detectable changes manifest [34]. Thus, molecular techniques like PCR, qPCR, and gene expression profiling are employed to identify genetic mutations or biomarkers linked to oral cancers at an early stage, enhancing prognosis [19, 35].

4.1.5 Diagnosis of hereditary disorders

Orodental disorders encompass a range of conditions affecting the dentition and oral cavity, including anomalies in tooth number, morphology, and size (e.g., selective tooth agenesis, microdontia, and globodontia), as well as structural defects (e.g., amelogenesis imperfecta, hereditary dentinogenesis imperfecta) and disturbances in tooth eruption. Numerous studies have elucidated the genetic etiology of these conditions, with mutations in genes such as PAX9, MSX1, WNT10A, and others identified as contributors to selective tooth agenesis (STHAG) [36]. Thus, molecular diagnostics like whole-genome sequencing (WGS) and next-generation sequencing (NGS) can be utilized to detect chromosomal abnormalities and inherited diseases by analyzing gene mutations, thereby contributing to the investigation of their underlying etiology [19, 37].

4.2 Treatment aspect

Molecular diagnostic testing plays a critical role in evaluating inherited and acquired genetic disorders and pharmacogenetic responses and in guiding diagnosis, prognosis, treatment strategies, and the identification of gene-specific therapeutic targets. Certain aspects are discussed in detail as follows:

4.2.1 Selection of appropriate antibiotic to treat drug-resistant bacterial infections

Molecular techniques such as PCR and microarray analysis involve the precise identification of antibiotic resistance genes or mutations in resistant strains, as well as the determination of the exact location of these genes [17]. Various mobile genetic elements, including plasmids, transposons, bacteriophages, integrons, and combinations of them, are notable nucleic acid targets for investigating the prevalence and spread of resistance genes in bacteria [38]. PCR can be employed to screen for antibiotic resistance genes within the microbial population linked to infection. This, in turn, ensures the use of the most appropriate and targeted antibiotic, improving treatment outcomes, reducing the risk of resistance, and minimizing the risk of treatment failure and unnecessary side effects from ineffective drugs. For instance, Evans SR et al. showed that rapid molecular diagnostic (RMD) platforms represent a valuable advancement in antimicrobial stewardship by enabling the swift and accurate identification of resistance determinants. These tools are particularly useful in guiding empiric β-lactam therapy when *bla* genes are not detected and local resistance patterns are well-characterized, thus supporting evidence-based selection of initial antimicrobial regimens and minimizing inappropriate antibiotic use [39].

4.2.2 Personalized treatment plans

PCR can offer valuable prognostic insights by assessing the severity and progression of these conditions based on the detected mutations. Personalized PCR-based therapies, customized to a patient's genetic profile, have the potential to optimize treatment results and reduce unwanted side effects [40].

For instance, dental caries susceptibility is estimated to be 40–60% heritable, with multiple genomic and locus-specific factors contributing to its pathogenesis. Variants in key genes—such as *AmelX*, involved in enamel biomineralization; *KLK4*, essential for enamel maturation; *LYZL2*, implicated in innate immune defense; and *AJAP1*, potentially influencing odontogenesis—have been associated with increased caries risk. The early identification of these genetic markers facilitates improved diagnostic precision and prognostic evaluation, enabling the implementation of personalized preventive and therapeutic strategies in clinical dentistry [41, 42].

Genetics is fundamental to understanding malocclusion and craniofacial anomalies in orthodontics. Conditions like Class III malocclusion and cleft lip and palate are strongly linked to specific genetic variants. For example, Class III malocclusion, seen in the Habsburg lineage, is often a monogenic dominant trait involving genes like *IHH*, *PTHLH*, *IGF1*, and *VEGF*. Cleft lip and palate are associated with genes such as *TMEM1*, *GAD1*, *IRF6*, *PVRL1*, and *MSX1*. Personalized orthodontics, driven by genetic profiling, enables early risk prediction and precise, individualized treatment strategies [43].

Genetic testing and molecular profiling allow for tailored treatments based on individual genetic makeup, determining the best approach for managing dental implants.

4.2.3 Monitoring of treatment efficacy

Molecular diagnostics can track the success of treatments, such as monitoring the bacterial load after periodontal therapy or checking the progression of oral diseases at the molecular level [44]. Specific biomarkers in peri-implant crevicular fluid (PICF) can indicate peri-implantitis, aiding in early detection and management of implant-related complications. Biomarkers like PGE2, sST2, CCL-20/MIP-3α, BAFF/BlyS, IL-23, RANKL, osteoprotegerin, and aMMP-8 have been studied for monitoring peri-implant health. PGE2 correlates with disease severity, while sST2 is linked to inflammation, such as periodontitis. IL-23 and RANKL help clarify the pathogenesis of peri-implant disease, highlighting the need for early diagnosis and monitoring [45, 46]. Molecular assays augment culture methods for detecting microorganisms in patients with prior antimicrobial treatment or when dealing with fastidious pathogens. Broad-range PCR targeting the 16S rRNA gene should be employed on culture-negative samples when infection is suspected based on clinical manifestations or inflammatory syndromes [47]. After dental implant placement, the biological processes involved in the integration of implants with cortical bone can be examined by analyzing the gene expression of osteoblasts (runx2, osteocalcin, collagen-I, and IGF-I) and osteoclasts (TRAP, H + -ATPase, and calcitonin receptor) through real-time reverse transcription PCR [48].

4.2.4 Treatment through optogenetics

Optogenetics is an innovative field that leverages light-responsive proteins, whose conformational changes upon light exposure initiate specific effects. This allows for precise control over gene activation or suppression. In dental medicine, it offers potential for tissue engineering, promoting cell differentiation, wound healing, and inhibiting malignant cells [49–51]. Niyazi M et al. [52] conducted an experiment in which human dental pulp stem cells (hDPSCs), isolated from an impacted third molar, were genetically modified to express the optogenetic actuator CaMKIIa-hChR2 (H134R) and exposed to 470 nm blue light stimulation over a five-day period. The results indicate that optogenetic stimulation enhances hDPSC viability and promotes their differentiation into neuron-like cells, underscoring its potential for application in regenerative therapies targeting neuronal repair [52].

4.2.5 Patient counseling

PCR-based genetic screening in dentistry is essential for genetic counseling in individuals and families with a predisposition to heritable dental disorders.

This method enables the precise identification of genetic variants that may elevate an individual's susceptibility to various oral diseases or conditions. By providing comprehensive insights into inheritance patterns—whether autosomal dominant, recessive, or X-linked—PCR screening helps assess the likelihood of these conditions being transmitted to offspring [40].

4.3 Preventive aspects

There is assured potential that the analysis of the genome, transcripts, and proteome can provide insight into what is occurring at a cellular level preceding the appearance of clinically observable change. Identifying genetic risk factors early allows for timely preventive measures, which can mitigate the onset of disease or reduce its severity. Thus, molecular techniques can assist in averting or minimizing the severity of the following conditions:

4.3.1 Oral disease and disorder prevention

i. Identifying high-risk individuals for dental caries: Molecular diagnostics can assess a person's likelihood of developing a disease, identify latent conditions, and thus help in the prevention and progression of the illness [22]. Genetic markers associated with an increased susceptibility to dental caries, periodontal diseases, and other oral health issues can be identified through PCR. Detecting these markers facilitates the creation of personalized prevention strategies [40]. For example, quantitative analysis of microbial load in saliva using quantitative PCR can help predict an individual's susceptibility to dental caries, as the microbial load of *Streptococcus mutans* and *Lactobacillus* in saliva is positively linked to the prevalence of dental caries [28].

ii. PCR-based genetic analysis to identify an individual's susceptibility to periodontitis can help guide the selection, frequency of treatment, and preventive measures for the disease [53]. Periodontitis is influenced by multiple genes, with at least 65 identified as being associated with the condition. Examining these genetic variations can help pinpoint individuals at greater risk, and various approaches for preventive treatment can be planned [54]. An available genetic test for severe chronic periodontitis detects two IL-1 alleles (IL-1α +4845 and IL-1β +3954). Individuals with both alleles are more likely to overexpress the gene, leading to elevated IL-1 levels in GCF and saliva, which increases the risk of severe periodontitis. Genomics thus helps predict periodontitis susceptibility in certain patients [55].

4.3.2 Systemic disease prevention

i. Certain oral diseases, like periodontitis, are associated with systemic conditions such as cardiovascular disease, diabetes, pregnancy, and perinatal complications. Timely detection with the help of molecular techniques and treatment of these oral diseases can help prevent the development of these related systemic health issues [56, 57].

ii. Genomic studies, such as DNA sequencing, can identify populations and individuals at higher risk, enabling them to take preventive measures and reduce their likelihood of developing the disease. Since PCR can detect mutations before clinical symptoms appear, it enables the early identification of genetic mutations linked to dental abnormalities. By analyzing DNA samples from individuals at risk, PCR can uncover these mutations ahead of time [40]. Furthermore, specific gene mutations associated with genetic oral conditions are often linked to systemic diseases. Early detection of mutations in relevant genes can prompt clinicians to monitor these patients regularly for potential systemic conditions, facilitating proactive management and intervention. For instance, mutations in the AXIN2 gene that cause Selective tooth agenesis (STHAG) have been shown to predispose carriers to colorectal cancer [58]. Early diagnosis of AXIN2 mutations can hence alert clinicians to counsel patients to have regular colonoscopies. Similarly, the identification of mutations in FAM20A in patients presenting with amelogenesis imperfecta can prompt a renal investigation for the management of nephrocalcinosis [59].

4.4 Research aspect: Impact of molecular techniques on dental research and clinical practice

Research is a crucial element in every field, fueling the creation of a diverse range of advanced tools. Through extensive studies, significant innovations—from molecular breakthroughs to advanced strategies tackling regenerative challenges in oral medicine—have been developed. Molecular technology, in particular, has proven to be a vital tool in this progress.

Dental research should be aligned with the oral health requirements of communities, a goal supported by advancements in technology. As biomedical technologies continue to progress, our understanding of vaccines, cloning, pharmaceuticals, DNA, tissues, microorganisms, viruses, and complex proteins is expanding swiftly, playing a key role in enhancing overall human health [60]. Numerous molecular methods, including PCR, gene expression analysis, microarrays, and others, have become essential research tools in the field of dentistry [19, 37]. Oral biofilm, a critical component of oral health, can be better understood through the use of molecular techniques [61].

The following areas present opportunities for further research.

4.4.1 Genetic research in dentistry

The study of oral tissue cell morphology, composition, and the genetic makeup of disorders can be further elucidated at the molecular level through advanced molecular techniques. These methods facilitate a deeper understanding of the genetic basis of various oral health conditions, including cleft lip and palate, tooth development disorders, and genetic predispositions to diseases such as gingivitis and periodontitis.

4.4.2 Research on the pathogenesis of orofacial diseases/disorders and their impact on systemic health

The study of oral pathogenetic mechanisms has been a central focus in oral biology research, with molecular diagnostics playing a crucial role in advancing our understanding of the link between oral and systemic complications. By enabling the detection and analysis of specific biomarkers, pathogens, and genetic alterations, molecular diagnostics enhances our ability to uncover these complex relationships.

This approach provides deeper insights into how oral health influences and contributes to the pathogenesis of systemic diseases [62, 63]. For example, *Fusobacterium nucleatum* (*F. nucleatum*), linked to periodontal disease, is more abundant near colorectal cancer lesions than in normal tissue. It promotes tumor growth by both enhancing cell proliferation and suppressing antitumor immunity. *F. nucleatum* interacts with the TIGIT receptor on natural killer cells via its Fap2 protein, inhibiting immune response and advancing colorectal cancer progression [64]. Genomics and proteomics can be used to investigate gene expression, offering important insights into the development of oral diseases such as granular cell tumors of the oral cavity [65, 66].

4.4.3 Studies to explore the role of microbes in oral cancer

Studies have indicated a link between periodontal disease and an increased risk of precancerous lesions and tumors [67]. Fungal infection with Candida has been linked to malignant oral development, notably causing oral leukoplakias and correlating with epithelial dysplasia [68]. As research on the relationship between the microbiome and carcinogenesis is still in its early stages, sequencing and PCR techniques can aid in uncovering many aspects that remain poorly understood.

4.4.4 Regenerative oral medicine

Molecular studies facilitate the understanding of the cellular mechanisms and signaling pathways governing the intrinsic regenerative potential of tissues, thereby advancing the exploration of novel guided tissue regeneration approaches that can be utilized for the repair of oral tissues [69]. Endogenous regenerative medicine (ERM) is an emerging field that harnesses the body's natural healing capacity by using it as an in vivo bioreactor to activate resident quiescent stem cells. This strategy presents a simpler, safer, and more cost-effective alternative to traditional exogenous approaches by promoting regeneration through targeted stem cell recruitment. In their review, Ivanov et al. highlight the potential of cell-free products—such as decellularized extracellular matrix, growth factors, extracellular vesicles, and miRNAs—in supporting endogenous bone and dental tissue regeneration [69]. Katagiri et al. conducted a pioneering clinical study to assess the safety and effectiveness of using conditioned medium derived from bone marrow mesenchymal stem cells (MSC-CM) for rebuilding alveolar bone in patients requiring augmentation before dental implants. The MSC-CM, enriched with bioactive molecules such as IGF-1, VEGF, TGF-β1, and HGF, was delivered using either β-tricalcium phosphate or atelocollagen scaffolds. The approach resulted in successful early bone formation, showed low inflammatory response, and had no adverse effects, indicating its strong potential as a regenerative treatment for bone repair [70].

4.4.5 Study of impact of different dental materials on oral tissue

Molecular technology can be used to analyze the properties of new dental materials, such as dental resin-based composites and dental alloys, and evaluate their interactions with oral tissues. Saini et al. conducted a study that addressed the challenges associated with adhesion and biomechanical properties in dental resin-based composites by employing both molecular docking and molecular dynamics (MDy) simulations. This approach was used to evaluate the interactions between the components and their effects on composite behavior. The study specifically focused on SiO_2 and (Trimethoxysilyl) propyl methacrylate (TRIS) due to their significant and consistent impact on composite properties. Furthermore, MDy simulations provided in-depth insights into the mechanical properties of dental composite complexes [71–73]. By examining factors such as biocompatibility, cellular response, cellular toxicity, local and systemic allergic effects, pulp reactions, estrogenic effects, and long-term stability, important factors can be determined using molecular techniques [74, 75]. This technology provides a deeper understanding of how these materials interact with oral tissues, promoting tissue regeneration, healing, and overall oral health [76]. This approach not only helps optimize material design but also ensures their safety and efficacy in clinical applications. Emerging concepts like bacteriophage therapy and nanoparticles, which target drug resistance, are gaining attention as potential solutions for combating oral microbial infections [77, 78]. To further investigate these areas, advanced techniques such as genetic sequencing can provide insights into the genetic composition of both the implicated bacteria and bacteriophages, thereby facilitating the identification of potentially therapeutic bacteriophages [79].

4.5 Forensic dentistry

Forensic odontology has become an integral part of forensic investigations [80]. Traditional investigative methods of forensic dentistry, such as dental records, X-rays, and bite marks, have proven valuable in human identification of the deceased in natural disasters, mass catastrophes, or crimes, and in examining sexual assault cases through bite mark analysis and dental age estimation [81].

In addition to the aforementioned traditional methods, molecular diagnostics have gained crucial attention in supporting forensic odontology. DNA evidence can be retrieved from traces of the perpetrator's saliva found in bite marks or indentations on the victim's body, aiding in the identification and confirmation of the suspect [81]. Furthermore, in specific cases, teeth are an essential source for genetic analysis and molecular studies, as they are resistant to post-mortem changes and environmental factors like extreme temperatures, physical trauma, and water submersion, making them a dependable source of DNA [82].

5. Future aspects

Molecular diagnostic techniques, despite their significant potential, are poised for further refinement to enhance their reliability and yield more precise and accurate results. Certain aspects that warrant further exploration are as follows:

5.1 Application of messenger RNA (mRNA) and ribosomal RNA (rRNA) in PCR

PCR techniques target bacterial fragments rather than viable, culturable cells, making it difficult to differentiate between live and dead microbes [6]. To enhance PCR accuracy and reduce false positives from bacterial genetic material in nonviable samples, targeting mRNA and rRNA can be more effective. These molecules degrade upon cell death, serving as reliable indicators of bacterial viability and accurately reflecting the living status of the bacteria [6, 83].

5.2 PCR amplification along with mass spectrometry

It enhances bacterial infection diagnosis by quantifying bacterial load and identifying bacterial species directly. This approach eliminates the need for lengthy DNA sequencing by leveraging mass spectrometry to analyze DNA fragment sequences and quantities. Melendez et al. demonstrated that the combination of PCR and electrospray ionization mass spectrometry (ESI-MS), when applied to synovial fluid specimens, achieved a diagnostic performance with 81% sensitivity and 95% specificity for the detection of prosthetic joint infections. A similar molecular approach may be employed to identify causative pathogens in oral infections, offering rapid and precise microbial diagnosis [84].

5.3 Droplet dPCR (ddPCR) application

Circular RNAs (circRNAs) are covalently closed, single-stranded RNAs with high stability and ubiquitous expression in eukaryotes. Their resistance to degradation and regulatory roles—such as sponging oncogenic microRNAs or interacting with proteins—make them promising biomarkers and therapeutic targets in cancer.

ddPCR is a highly sensitive and precise method for absolute quantification of nucleic acids, particularly effective for low-abundance targets like circRNAs. The technique partitions samples into ~20,000 nanoliter-sized droplets, each undergoing individual PCR amplification. Fluorescence-based detection enables accurate quantification based on Poisson statistics. ddPCR, a highly sensitive variant of PCR, can be used to detect and quantify these biomarkers, aiding in the diagnosis and prognosis of oral cancers [85].

5.4 Artificial intelligence (AI) and molecular diagnostics

In the contemporary medical landscape, AI has emerged as a transformative tool, particularly in diagnostics and precision medicine. One of its most impactful applications in clinical genomics is the extraction and integration of high-resolution phenotypic data from diverse sources such as medical imaging, electronic health records (EHRs), and biomedical devices. This capability enhances genomic analysis by enabling more accurate variant detection, genome annotation, and prediction of the functional consequences of genetic alterations. When combined with molecular diagnostics, AI facilitates the development of personalized treatment strategies by allowing clinicians to assess disease risk, identify therapeutic targets, and tailor interventions based on an individual's unique genetic profile [86, 87].

In dentistry, machine learning (ML)—a subset of AI—is increasingly used to analyze complex datasets derived from diagnostic modalities such as radiographs, cone-beam computed tomography (CBCT), and intraoral imaging. These algorithms enhance diagnostic accuracy for conditions including dental caries, periodontal disease, and oral malignancies, while reducing inter-observer variability and streamlining clinical decision-making.

Beyond diagnostics, ML enhances personalized dental care by predicting treatment outcomes based on factors like bone density, oral microbiota, and patient behavior. Combined with 3D printing, ML enables the creation of customized prosthetics and orthodontic devices.

The integration of optogenetics and ML marks a novel advance in dental research. ML can analyze data from optogenetic studies on orofacial pain to build predictive models and optimize stimulation parameters for targeted cellular responses. This synergy offers promising potential for personalized neuromodulatory therapies and precision-driven dental care [88].

6. Discussion

Molecular diagnostics has introduced transformative possibilities in dentistry, yet its integration into routine clinical practice faces notable limitations. Chief among these are the high costs of implementation, technical complexity, and the need for specialized infrastructure and personnel. These barriers restrict access, particularly in general dental settings and underserved regions. Moreover, many identified biomarkers have not undergone rigorous, large-scale validation, raising concerns about their reproducibility and reliability in diverse patient populations.

Ethical and psychosocial considerations further complicate the use of genetic screening in preventive dental care. Communicating genetic risks can be challenging, especially when patients have limited health literacy or lack contextual understanding of probabilistic information. This may lead to anxiety, misinformed choices, or unnecessary interventions. In parallel, regulatory oversight for advanced tools such as next-generation sequencing (NGS) remains inconsistent across jurisdictions, contributing to variability in data interpretation, clinical reporting, and overall diagnostic quality.

Despite these hurdles, molecular diagnostics continues to expand the frontiers of oral healthcare. Genomics enables the detection of hereditary mutations and oncogenic changes, while proteomics and metabolomics offer insights into disease-specific biomarkers and metabolic dysfunctions seen in conditions like oral cancer, periodontitis, and developmental disorders. Techniques such as PCR and NGS facilitate early diagnosis, microbial profiling, and risk stratification—enabling more timely and personalized treatment strategies.

In research, these molecular approaches have accelerated progress in regenerative dentistry, particularly in stem cell-based therapies and biomaterial-guided tissue repair, though most remain in experimental or early translational stages. Forensic dentistry also benefits, with DNA extracted from teeth and bite marks serving as robust and durable evidence in human identification, even under extreme post-mortem conditions.

Emerging technologies such as AI are beginning to bridge the gap between molecular diagnostics and clinical practice. AI-powered platforms can analyze large, complex molecular datasets rapidly and with high accuracy, improving diagnostic efficiency and biomarker discovery. Furthermore, AI can assist in integrating genomic, proteomic, and clinical data to support predictive modeling, risk assessment, and decision-making. As molecular diagnostics and AI evolve in parallel, their convergence promises to transform dentistry into a more precise, predictive, and personalized discipline—paving the way for a future of smarter, data-driven oral healthcare.

7. Conclusion

In conclusion, molecular diagnostics is transforming modern dentistry by enabling the precise detection and analysis of genetic makeup, pathogens, and biomarkers in oral tissues. It enhances our understanding of the underlying causes and progression of oromaxillofacial conditions, paving the way for more precise diagnoses and targeted therapies. With the application of advanced techniques like PCR and next-generation sequencing, molecular diagnostics enhances early detection, facilitates personalized care, and ultimately improves patient outcomes. As this field continues to evolve, it holds the potential to revolutionize both preventive and therapeutic practices in dentistry, fostering a new era of precision oral healthcare.

Acknowledgements

The authors thank their family members and colleagues for their support and the Institute of Medical Sciences, Banaras Hindu University, for providing the resources. They also acknowledge the use of Artificial Intelligence tools for language polishing of the manuscript. Microsoft Office PowerPoint was used to create figures.

Conflict of interest

None.

Author details

Gopal Nath and Alka Shukla*
Viral Research and Diagnostic Laboratory, Department of Microbiology, Faculty of Medicine, Institute of Medical Sciences, Banaras Hindu University, Varanasi, UP, India

*Address all correspondence to: alka.vrdl@gmail.com

References

[1] Ahmad P, Rubbia Nawaz MQ, Shaikh GM, Mohamed RN, Nagarajappa AK, Asif JA, et al. Risk factors associated with the mortality rate of oral squamous cell carcinoma patients: A 10-year retrospective study. Medicine. 2021;**100**:e27127

[2] Wu L, Zhang SQ, Zhao L, Ren ZH, Hu CY. Global, regional, and national burden of periodontitis from 1990 to 2019: Results from the global burden of disease study 2019. Journal of Periodontology. 2022;**93**(10):1445-1454

[3] Debnath M, Prasad GB, Bisen PS. Molecular Diagnostics: Promises and Possibilities. Netherlands: Springer Netherlands; 2010

[4] Braziel RM, Shipp MA, Feldman AL, Espina V, Winters M, Jaffe ES, et al. Molecular diagnostics. Hematology. American Society of Hematology. Education Program. 2003;(1):279-293

[5] Brown ZJ, Patwardhan S, Bean J, Pawlik TM. Molecular diagnostics and biomarkers in cholangiocarcinoma. Surgical Oncology. 2022;**44**:101851

[6] Choe H, Deirmengian CA, Hickok NJ, Morrison TN, Tuan RS. Molecular diagnostics. The Journal of the American Academy of Orthopaedic Surgeons. 2015;**23 Suppl**:S26-S31

[7] Hocquette JF. Where are we in genomics? Journal of Physiology and Pharmacology. 2005 Jun;**1**(56):37

[8] McArdle AJ, Menikou S. What is proteomics? Archives of Disease in Childhood. Education and Practice Edition. 2021;**106**(3):178-181

[9] Lawrance IC, Klopcic B, Wasinger VC. Proteomics: An overview. Inflammatory Bowel Diseases. 2005;**11**(10):927-936

[10] Clish CB. Metabolomics: An emerging but powerful tool for precision medicine. Cold Spring Harbor Molecular Case Studies. 2015;**1**(1):a000588

[11] Gerszten RE, Wang TJ. The search for new cardiovascular biomarkers. Nature. 2008;**451**:949-952

[12] Serkova NJ, Spratlin JL, Eckhardt SG. NMR-based metabolomics: Translational application and treatment of cancer. Current Opinion in Molecular Therapeutics. 2007;**9**(6):572-585

[13] Bartella L, Thakur SB, Morris EA, et al. Enhancing nonmass lesions in the breast: Evaluation with proton (1H) MR spectroscopy. Radiology. 2007;**245**(1):80-87

[14] Patil S, Rao RS, Sanketh DS, Amrutha N. Microbial flora in oral diseases. The Journal of Contemporary Dental Practice. 2013;**14**(6):1202

[15] Socransky SS, Haffajee AD. Periodontal microbial ecology. Periodontology 2000. 2000;**2005**(38):135-187

[16] Booth V, Downes J, Van den Berg J, Wade WG. Gram-positive anaerobic bacilli in human periodontal disease. Journal of Periodontal Research. 2004;**39**(4):213-220

[17] Aarts HJM, Guerra B, Malorny B. Molecular methods for detection of antimicrobial resistance. In: Antimicrobial Resistance in Bacteria of Animal Origin. Washington, DC, USA: ASM Press; 2006

[18] Zhang S, Li X, Wu J, Coin L, O'Brien J, Hai F, et al. Molecular methods for pathogenic bacteria detection and

recent advances in wastewater analysis. Water. 2021;**13**(24):3551

[19] Vaid NCP, Bansal P, Bhargava K, Bhargava D. Polymerase chain reaction & its applications in dentistry. European Journal of Pharmaceutical and Medical Research. 2016;**3**(12):185-189

[20] Reynolds SJ, Muwonga J. OraQuick advance rapid HIV-1/2 antibody test. Expert Review of Molecular Diagnostics. 2004;**4**(5):587-591

[21] Shukla A, Gangwar M, Sharma G, Prakash P, Nath G. Vitality of proteinase K in rRTPCR detection of SARS-CoV2 bypassing RNA extraction. Frontiers in Cellular and Infection Microbiology. 2021;**11**:717068

[22] Dwivedi S, Purohit P, Misra R, Pareek P, Goel A, Khattri S, et al. Diseases and molecular diagnostics: A step closer to precision medicine. Indian Journal of Clinical Biochemistry. 2017;**32**(4):374-398

[23] Ebersole JL, Nagarajan R, Akers D, Miller CS. Targeted salivary biomarkers for discrimination of periodontal health and disease(s). Frontiers in Cellular and Infection Microbiology. 2015;**5**:6

[24] Lahteenmaki H, Umeizudike KA, Heikkinen AM, et al. aMMP-8 point-of-care/chairside oral fluid technology as a rapid, non-invasive tool for periodontitis and peri-implantitis screening in a medical care setting. Diagnostics. 2020;**10**:562

[25] Golub LM, Räisänen IT, Sorsa T, Preshaw PM. An unexplored pharmacologic/diagnostic strategy for peri-implantitis: A protocol proposal. Diagnostics. 2020;**10**:1050

[26] Bornes R, Montero J, Correia A, et al. Peri-implant diseases diagnosis, prognosis and dental implant monitoring: A narrative review of novel strategies and clinical impact. BMC Oral Health. 2023;**23**(1):183

[27] Zhang A, Sun H, Wang X. Saliva metabolomics opens door to biomarker discovery, disease diagnosis, and treatment. Applied Biochemistry and Biotechnology. 2012;**168**:1718-1727

[28] Zhang CZ, Cheng XQ, Li JY, Zhang P, Yi P, Xu X, et al. Saliva in the diagnosis of diseases. International Journal of Oral Science. 2016;**8**(3):133-137

[29] Engebretson SP, Grbic JT, Singer R, Lamster IB. GCF IL-1-beta profiles in periodontal disease. Journal of Clinical Periodontology. 2002;**29**(1):48-53

[30] Rathnayake N, Akerman S, Klinge B, et al. Salivary biomarkers for detection of systemic diseases. PLoS One. 2013;**8**(4):e61356

[31] McGurk M, Chan C, Jones J, O'Regan E, Sherriff M. Delay in diagnosis and its effect on outcome in head and neck cancer. The British Journal of Oral & Maxillofacial Surgery. 2005;**43**(4):281-284

[32] Hadzic S, Gojkov-Vukelic M, Pasic E, Dervisevic A. Importance of early detection of potentially malignant lesions in the prevention of oral cancer. Materia Socio-Medica. 2017;**29**(2):129

[33] Sciubba JJ. Oral cancer: The importance of early diagnosis and treatment. American Journal of Clinical Dermatology. 2001;**2**:239-251

[34] Yap T, Celentano A, Seers C, McCullough MJ, Farah CS. Molecular diagnostics in oral cancer and oral potentially malignant disorders—A clinician's guide. Journal of Oral Pathology & Medicine. 2020;**49**(1):1-8

[35] Ford PJ, Farah CS. Early detection and diagnosis of oral cancer: Strategies for improvement. Journal of Cancer Policy. 2013;**1**(1-2):e2-e7

[36] Prasad MK, Geoffroy V, Vicaire S, et al. A targeted next-generation sequencing assay for the molecular diagnosis of genetic disorders with orodental involvement. Journal of Medical Genetics. 2016;**53**(2):98-110

[37] Güven Y. Scientific basis of dentistry. Journal of Istanbul University Faculty of Dentistry. 2017;**51**(3):64-71

[38] Rizzo L, Manaia C, Merlin C, Schwartz T, Dagot C, Ploy MC, et al. Urban wastewater treatment plants as hotspots for antibiotic resistant bacteria and genes spread into the environment: A review. Science of the Total Environment. 2013;**447**:345-360

[39] Evans SR, Hujer AM, Jiang H, Hujer KM, Hall T, Marzan C, et al. Rapid molecular diagnostics, antibiotic treatment decisions, and developing approaches to inform empiric therapy: PRIMERS I and II. Clinical Infectious Diseases. 2016;**62**(2):181-189

[40] Khan N, Haque MI, Shenoy S, Puthenkandathil R, Kale P. Molecular dentistry: Polymerase chain reaction's transformative role. Journal of Cellular Biotechnology. 2024;**10**(1):101-107

[41] Eng G, Chen A, Vess T, Ginsburg GS. Genome technologies and personalized dental medicine. Oral Diseases. 2012;**18**(3):223-235

[42] Shaffer JR, Feingold E, Wang X, Lee M, Tcuenco K, Weeks DE, et al. GWAS of dental caries patterns in the permanent dentition. Journal of Dental Research. 2013;**92**(1):38-44

[43] Reddy MS, Shetty SR, Vannala V. Embracing personalized medicine in dentistry. Journal of Pharmacy & Bioallied Sciences. 2019;**11**(Suppl 2):S92-S96

[44] Ramseier CA. Diagnostic measures for monitoring and follow-up in periodontology and implant dentistry. Periodontology 2000. 2024;**95**(1):129-155

[45] Lang NP, Berglundh T. Working group 4 of seventh European workshop on periodontology. Periimplant diseases: Where are we now? – Consensus of the seventh European workshop on periodontology. Journal of Clinical Periodontology. 2011;**38**(Suppl 11):178-181

[46] Ramanauskaite A, Juodzbalys G. Diagnostic principles of peri-implantitis: A systematic review and guidelines for peri-implantitis diagnosis proposal. Journal of Oral & Maxillofacial Research. 2016;**7**:e8

[47] Lévy PY, Fenollar F. The role of molecular diagnostics in implant-associated bone and joint infection. Clinical Microbiology and Infection. 2012;**18**(12):1168-1175

[48] Monjo M, Lamolle SF, Lyngstadaas SP, Rønold HJ, Ellingsen JE. In vivo expression of osteogenic markers and bone mineral density at the surface of fluoride-modified titanium implants. Biomaterials. 2008;**29**(28):3771-3780

[49] Steinberg T, Dieterle MP, Tomakidi P. Molecular research on oral diseases and related biomaterials: A journey from oral cell models to advanced regenerative perspectives. International Journal of Molecular Sciences. 2022;**23**(9):5288

[50] Huang D, Li R, Ren J, Luo H, Wang W, Zhou C. Temporal induction of Lhx8 by optogenetic control system for efficient bone regeneration. Stem Cell Research & Therapy. 2021;**12**:339

[51] Spagnuolo G, Genovese F, Fortunato L, Simeone M, Rengo C, Tatullo M. The impact of optogenetics on regenerative medicine. Applied Sciences. 2019;**10**:173

[52] Niyazi M, Zibaii MI, Chavoshinezhad S, Hamidabadi HG, Dargahi L, Bojnordi MN, et al. Neurogenic differentiation of human dental pulp stem cells by optogenetics stimulation. Journal of Chemical Neuroanatomy. 2020;**109**:101821

[53] Maheaswari R, Kshirsagar JT, Lavanya N. Polymerase chain reaction: A molecular diagnostic tool in periodontology. Journal of Indian Society of Periodontology. 2016;**20**(2):128-135

[54] Loos BG, Van Dyke TE. The role of inflammation and genetics in periodontal disease. Periodontology 2000. 2020;**83**:26-39

[55] Taba M Jr, Kinney J, Kim AS, Giannobile WV. Diagnostic biomarkers for oral and periodontal diseases. Dental Clinics of North America. 2005;**49**(3):551-571

[56] Dolińska E, Wiśniewski P, Pietruska M. Periodontal molecular diagnostics: State of knowledge and future prospects for clinical application. International Journal of Molecular Sciences. 2024;**25**(23):12624

[57] Usui M, Onizuka S, Sato T, Kokabu S, Ariyoshi W, Nakashima K. Mechanism of alveolar bone destruction in periodontitis — Periodontal bacteria and inflammation. Journal of Dental Sciences. 2021;**57**:201-208

[58] Lammi L, Arte S, Somer M, Järvinen H, Lahermo P, Thesleff I, et al. Mutations in AXIN2 cause familial tooth agenesis and predispose to colorectal cancer. American Journal of Human Genetics. 2004;**74**:1043-1050

[59] de La Dure-Molla M, Quentric M, Yamaguti PM, Acevedo A-C, Mighell AJ, Vikkula M, et al. Pathognomonic oral profile of enamel renal syndrome (ERS) caused by recessive FAM20A mutations. Orphanet Journal of Rare Diseases. 2014;**9**:84

[60] Ford P, Seymour G, Beeley JA, Curro F, Depaola D, Ferguson D, et al. Adapting to changes in molecular biosciences and technologies. European Journal of Dental Education. 2008;**12**(Suppl 1):40-47

[61] Hiyari S, Bennett KM. Dental diagnostics: Molecular analysis of oral biofilms. The Journal of Dental Hygiene Association. 2011;**85**(4):256-263

[62] Yoshida RA, Lobato TB, Gorjão R, França LS, Alves LA, Santos MTBR. Detection and quantification of pathogens in saliva of adolescents with cerebral palsy: A cross-sectional study. Frontiers in Dental Medicine. 2023;**4**:1208243

[63] Xiao X, Liu S, Deng H, Song Y, Zhang L, Song Z. Advances in the oral microbiota and rapid detection of oral infectious diseases. Frontiers in Microbiology. 2023;**14**:1121737

[64] Goto T. Microbiota and lung cancer. Seminars in Cancer Biology. 2022;**86**(3):1-10

[65] Rogala B, Khan ZA, Jackson-Boeters L, Darling MR. Investigation of the molecular profile of granular cell tumours and schwannomas of the oral cavity. Dental Journal. 2022;**10**(3):38

[66] McDaniel S, McDaniel J, Howard KM, Kingsley K. Molecular screening and analysis reveal novel oral site-specific locations for the cariogenic pathogen Scardoviawiggsiae. Dental Journal. 2021;**9**(6):73

[67] Tezal M, Grossi SG, Genco RJ. Is periodontitis associated with oral neoplasms? Journal of Periodontology. 2005;**76**(3):406-410

[68] Hooper SJ, Wilson MJ, Crean SJ. Exploring the link between microorganisms and oral cancer: A systematic review of the literature. Head & Neck. 2009;**31**(9):1228-1239

[69] Ivanov AA, Kuznetsova AV, Popova OP, Danilova TI, Yanushevich OO. Modern approaches to acellular therapy in bone and dental regeneration. International Journal of Molecular Sciences. 2021;**22**(24):13454

[70] Katagiri W, Osugi M, Kawai T, Hibi H. First-in-human study and clinical case reports of the alveolar bone regeneration with the secretome from human mesenchymal stem cells. Head & Face Medicine. 2016;**12**:5

[71] Schmalz G, Arenholt-Bindslev D. Biocompatibility of Dental Materials. Berlin: Springer; 2009

[72] Saini RS, Binduhayyim RI, Gurumurthy V, Alshadidi AA, Aldosari LI, Okshah A, et al. Dental biomaterials redefined: Molecular docking and dynamics-driven dental resin composite optimization. BMC Oral Health. 2024;**24**(1):557

[73] Nawrocka A, Piwonski I, Sauro S, Porcelli A, Hardan L, Lukomska-Szymanska M. Traditional microscopic techniques employed in dental adhesion research—Applications and protocols of specimen preparation. Biosensors. 2021;**11**(11):408

[74] Bakopoulou A, Papadopoulos T, Garefis P. Molecular toxicology of substances released from resin-based dental restorative materials. International Journal of Molecular Sciences. 2009;**10**(9):3861-3899

[75] Rosa V, Silikas N, Yu B, Dubey N, Sriram G, Zinelis S, et al. Guidance on the assessment of biocompatibility of biomaterials: Fundamentals and testing considerations. Dental Materials. 2024;**40**(11):1773-1785

[76] Meto A, Meto A. Evaluation of dental materials and oral disease-related proteins in dentistry: Efficacy of electrophoresis as a valuable tool. In: Electrophoresis-Recent Advances, New Perspectives and Applications. London, UK: IntechOpen; 2023

[77] Shukla A, Sharma S, Gangwar M, Sharma G, Rao BA. Association and contribution of dentistry in creating and sharing the burden of antibiotic-resistant microbial world. In: Emerging Paradigms for Antibiotic-Resistant Infections: Beyond the Pill. Singapore: Springer Nature Singapore; 2024. pp. 295-311

[78] Gangwar M, Rastogi S, Singh D, Shukla A, Dhameja N, Kumar D, et al. Immunological and safety profile of bacteriophage therapy: A preclinical study. Journal of Applied Microbiology. 2022;**133**(3):1446-1460

[79] Lima-Mendez G, Toussaint A, Leplae R. Analysis of the phage sequence space: The benefit of structured information. Virology. 2007;**365**(2):241-249

[80] da Silva RF, Pereira SD, Júnior ED, Barcelos RD, Godinho NM, Souto R. Genetics and molecular biology: A literature review of forensic dentistry application. Brazilian Journal of Oral Sciences. 2016;**6**(20):1254-1259

[81] Malik SD, Pillai JP, Malik U. Forensic genetics: Scope and application from forensic odontology perspective. Journal

of Oral and Maxillofacial Pathology. 2022;**26**(4):558-563

[82] Schwartz TR, Schwartz EA, Mieszerski L, McNally L, Kobilinsky L. Characterization of deoxyribonucleic acid (DNA) obtained from teeth subjected to various environmental conditions. Journal of Forensic Sciences. 1991;**36**:979-990

[83] Bergin PF, Doppelt JD, Hamilton WG, et al. Detection of periprosthetic infections with use of ribosomal RNA-based polymerase chain reaction. The Journal of Bone and Joint Surgery. American Volume. 2010;**92**(3):654-663

[84] Melendez DP, Uhl JR, Greenwood-Quaintance KE, Hanssen AD, Sampath R, Patel R. Detection of prosthetic joint infection by use of PCR-electrospray ionization mass spectrometry applied to synovial fluid. Journal of Clinical Microbiology. 2014;**52**(6):2202-2205

[85] Peng J, Li F, Xu X, Hu S. Single-cell analysis of circRNA using ddPCR. Methods in Molecular Biology. 2023;**2689**:169-177

[86] Li H, Xu H, Li Y, Li X. Application of artificial intelligence (AI)-enhanced biochemical sensing in molecular diagnosis and imaging analysis: Advancing and challenges. TrAC Trends in Analytical Chemistry. 2024;**174**:117700

[87] Dias R, Torkamani A. Artificial intelligence in clinical and genomic diagnostics. Genome Medicine. 2019;**11**(1):70

[88] Murugan R. Leveraging optogenetics and machine learning for precision dentistry. British Dental Journal. 2025;**238**:210

Chapter 3

Advancements in Molecular Diagnostics for Viral Outbreaks: A Focus on Respiratory Virus

Santiago Saavedra-Alonso, Ana Karina Chávez-Escamilla, Brenda Leticia Escobedo-Guajardo, Genoveva Alvarez-Ojeda, Carlos Alberto González-Villarreal, María Guadalupe Moreno-Treviño and Juan Francisco Lugo-Ibarra

Abstract

Human interaction with natural ecosystems, such as deforestation and animal markets, increases the risk of the emergence of new zoonotic viruses. Added to this is the constant mutation of already existing viruses, such as influenza, which can trigger new epidemics. Additionally, climate change alters animal migration patterns, thus facilitating the spread of infectious diseases. Among the recent outbreaks of viral respiratory diseases, the most notable are COVID-19 (SARS-CoV-2), which emerged in 2019 in Wuhan, China; the H1N1 swine influenza pandemic, which appeared in 2009 in Mexico; and avian flu, caused by the AH5N1 and AH7N9 influenza viruses, recorded since 1997 with limited transmission from birds to humans. Other outbreaks include AH3N2 and AH5N6, which have emerged since 2016, causing isolated cases with symptoms like seasonal influenza. Furthermore, within the other coronavirus family, notable mentions include MERS, which appeared in 2012 in Saudi Arabia, and SARS, which emerged in 2002 in China. In general, these respiratory diseases share similar symptoms, ranging from fever and cough to severe pneumonia, making their diagnosis and epidemiological monitoring challenging. For this reason, this chapter will thoroughly address the molecular diagnosis of respiratory diseases as a key tool for the identification and clinical management of these infections.

Keywords: quantitative PCR, next-generation sequencing, MXene-based biosensors, influenza, COVID-19

1. Introduction

Recent advancements in molecular diagnostics have significantly enhanced our ability to detect and manage viral outbreaks, particularly those involving respiratory viruses. Acute infectious respiratory diseases, affecting the ears, nose, throat, and lungs, pose a global health challenge due to their high morbidity and mortality rates in both children and adults.

These diseases are primarily caused by viruses, although bacteria, fungi, and parasites, and the symptoms often overlap, complicating accurate diagnosis in routine clinical practice. Therefore, precise molecular diagnostic techniques are crucial for:

- Optimizing patient management.
- Reducing unnecessary antibiotic use, especially for nonbacterial infections.
- Implementing specific antiviral treatments when available.
- Minimizing unnecessary diagnostic tests.
- Adopting public health measures to contain the spread of infections.
- Controlling potential outbreaks within and outside hospital settings.

Traditionally, diagnostic tests were confined to centralized laboratories due to the need for specialized equipment and trained personnel. However, recent innovations include point-of-care testing (POCT), which allows diagnostics to be performed in various settings such as homes, healthcare offices, emergency departments, and even space shuttles.

While laboratory-based tests remain the gold standard for their specificity and sensitivity, POCT offers rapid and accessible alternatives. Both methods are evaluated using receiver operating characteristic (ROC) curves, which assess their sensitivity and specificity, crucial for distinguishing between infected and healthy individuals.

In summary, the integration of advanced molecular diagnostics into routine practice is pivotal for improving outbreak response and patient outcomes in respiratory viral infections.

2. Traditional tests for the diagnosis of respiratory diseases

Respiratory infections are a significant public health concern, with various diagnostic methods employed to identify the causative pathogens. Traditional laboratory diagnostics include virus culture, antigen detection, enzyme-linked immunosorbent assay, serological methods, and fluorescence detection. Each of these methods has its strengths and limitations, which are critical for accurate diagnosis and management of respiratory infections.

2.1 Virus culture

Virus culture has long been considered the gold standard for diagnosing viral respiratory infections. This method involves isolating the virus from clinical specimens, allowing for the identification of specific pathogens. For instance, studies have shown that human bronchial epithelial cells (HBTEC-ALI), as described in **Figure 1A**, are particularly effective for isolating respiratory viruses due to their broad susceptibility to various pathogens [1]. However, virus culture can be

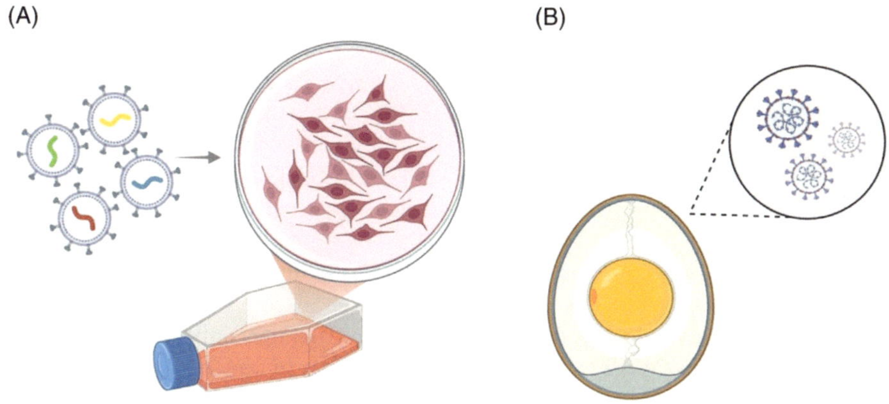

Figure 1.
Scheme of viral culture. (A) Viral culture in eukaryotic cells and (B) Viral culture in embryonated eggs. Source: This image is the author's original work and was created using the BioRender application.

time-consuming and may not always yield results, especially for viruses that require specific growth conditions, for example, culture in embryonated eggs as described in **Figure 1B**, or are present in low quantities [2]. Moreover, the cytopathic effects observed in cell cultures can sometimes be misleading, necessitating further confirmatory tests [3].

2.2 The enzyme-linked immunosorbent assay (ELISA) and immunochromatographic arrays

The enzyme-linked immunosorbent assay and immunochromatographic arrays are two prevalent immunoassay techniques utilized for the detection of various analytes, including proteins, pathogens, and toxins. Both methods have unique advantages and limitations, making them suitable for different applications in clinical diagnostics, food safety, and environmental monitoring.

Enzyme-linked immunosorbent assay is a widely recognized method that employs enzyme-linked antibodies to detect specific antigens in a sample, as described in **Figure 2A**. It is characterized by its high sensitivity and specificity, making it suitable for quantifying low concentrations of analytes. For instance, studies have shown

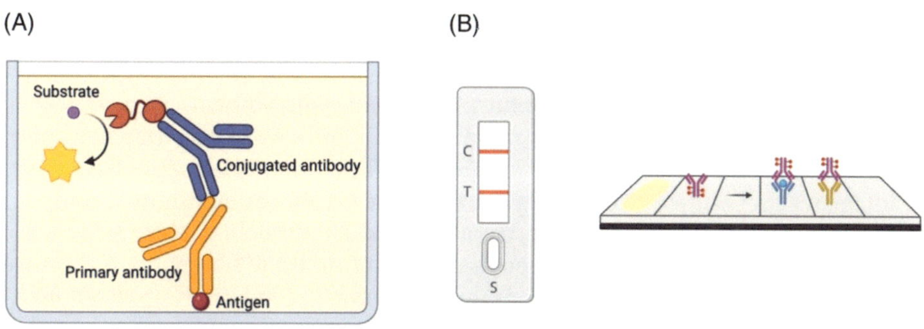

Figure 2.
(A) Scheme of ELISA and (B) Immunochromatographic arrays. Source: This image is the author's original work and was created using the BioRender application.

that ELISA can achieve sensitivities of up to 91% for detecting antibodies against various pathogens, such as the porcine reproductive and respiratory syndrome virus [4]. Furthermore, advancements in ELISA technology, such as the development of single-molecule ELISA, have enabled the detection of serum proteins at subfemtomolar concentrations, significantly enhancing its analytical capabilities [5]. However, traditional ELISA methods often require complex sample preparation and are time-consuming, which can limit their utility in point-of-care settings [6].

2.2.1 Development of ELISA innovations for SARS-CoV-2 and influenza A

Recent innovations in ELISA technology have significantly enhanced the sensitivity and speed of SARS-CoV-2 and influenza testing, largely due to the development of automated and optimized assays. For SARS-CoV-2, new automated bead-based immunoassays and cell-based ELISA techniques, such as IceLisa, have emerged, allowing for the rapid quantification of neutralizing antibodies (NABs) without requiring complex laboratory setups. This advancement accelerates the testing process [7, 8]. Moreover, adaptive orthogonal testing strategies have been implemented, combining multiple assays to improve specificity while maintaining high sensitivity, achieving up to 100% specificity with minimal loss in sensitivity [9]. Additionally, receptor-binding domain (RBD)-based ELISAs have demonstrated promising results, with sensitivity rates reaching 92.14% in symptomatic individuals, indicating a strong immune response to vaccination or infection [10]. Together, these advancements contribute to more efficient and reliable SARS-CoV-2 antibody testing, which is essential for monitoring immunity and informing public health strategies.

For influenza virus detection, the use of positively charged gold nanoparticles (+Au NPs) as inorganic peroxidase-mimicking enzymes in a modified ELISA has exhibited a 500-fold increase in sensitivity compared to commercial virus kits, effectively detecting clinically isolated influenza A (H1N1) and influenza A (H3N2) in complex biological samples [11]. Additionally, a rapid ELISA method has been developed that enhances test throughput by conducting initial reactions in a homogeneous phase, reducing the total testing time from up to 5 hours to under 30 minutes. This improvement makes the method more suitable for automation and high-throughput applications [12]. Furthermore, the use of fluorescently doped silica nanoparticles in lateral flow immunoassays (LFIAs) has resulted in an 8-fold increase in sensitivity compared to traditional gold nanoparticle-based systems, allowing for the detection of influenza nucleoprotein A at concentrations as low as 250 ng/ml within just 30 minutes [13]. These advancements not only enhance the sensitivity and speed of influenza A detection but also facilitate the integration of these assays into automated and portable diagnostic platforms, thereby broadening their applicability in both clinical and field settings.

In contrast, immunochromatographic assays, commonly known as lateral flow tests, as described in **Figure 2B**, offer rapid and straightforward detection methods that can yield results in as little as 15–20 minutes. These assays are particularly advantageous for point-of-care testing due to their ease of use and minimal equipment requirements [14]. For example, a multiplexed immunochromatographic strip has been developed for the simultaneous detection of multiple staphylococcal enterotoxins, demonstrating the potential for rapid screening in food safety applications [15]. Additionally, the integration of gold nanoparticles in immunochromatographic assays enhances sensitivity and allows for visual detection of analytes [16]. However, while these tests provide quick results, they may lack the quantitative precision and sensitivity of ELISA, particularly for low-abundance targets [17].

Recent innovations in both techniques have aimed to improve their performance. For instance, the use of nanomaterials, such as gold nanoparticles and silver nanoclusters, has been explored to enhance the sensitivity of immunochromatographic assays [18]. Similarly, the development of multiplexed formats in both ELISA and immunochromatographic assays allows for the simultaneous detection of multiple analytes, which is particularly beneficial in complex sample matrices like food or clinical specimens [19, 20]. These advancements highlight the ongoing evolution of immunoassay technologies to meet the increasing demand for rapid, sensitive, and specific detection methods across various fields.

2.3 Serological and antigen detection

Serological methods, including the detection of antibodies against specific respiratory pathogens, as described in **Figure 3A** and **B**, play a crucial role in diagnosing infections, particularly in cases where acute viral infections are suspected. These methods can help identify past infections and assess immune responses, which is particularly important in pediatric populations [21]. However, serological tests often require a second sample for comparison, as described in **Figure 3B**, which can delay diagnosis and treatment [22]. Additionally, the presence of antibodies does not always correlate with active infection, necessitating caution in interpretation [23].

Antigen detection tests provide a rapid means of diagnosing respiratory infections by identifying viral proteins in clinical samples. These tests are particularly useful in acute settings where timely diagnosis is crucial. For example, immunofluorescence assays have demonstrated high sensitivity and specificity for detecting respiratory viruses such as respiratory syncytial virus (RSV) and influenza [24]. However, the accuracy of antigen detection can be influenced by the timing of sample collection and the viral load present in the specimen, which may lead to false negatives [25].

2.4 Immunofluorescence detection

Fluorescence detection techniques, such as multiplex PCR assays, have revolutionized the diagnosis of respiratory infections by allowing for the simultaneous detection of multiple pathogens in a single test. These methods have been shown to improve diagnostic accuracy and reduce the time to diagnosis, which is critical in managing respiratory infections [26]. However, the complexity of these assays and the need for

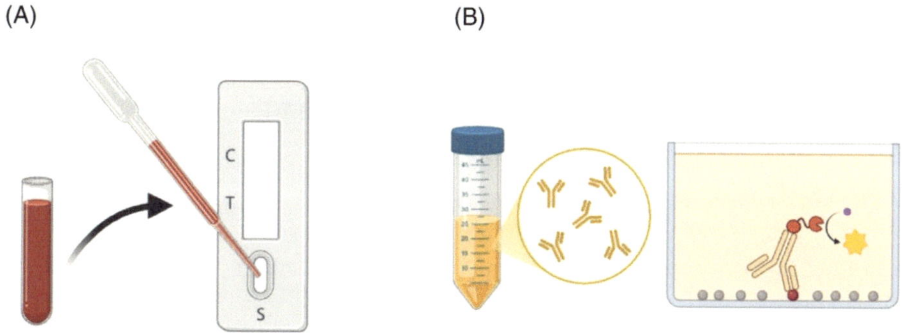

Figure 3.
Scheme of serological diagnosis from (A) whole blood or (B) serum. Source: This image is the author's original work and was created using the BioRender application.

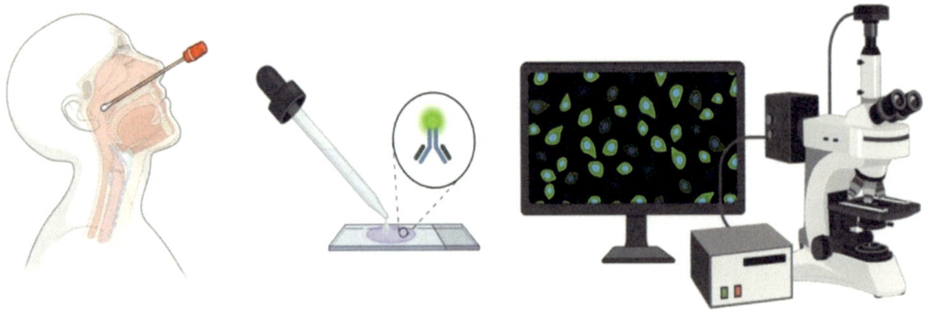

Figure 4.
Schematic diagram of the collection and observation of samples by direct immunofluorescence. Source: This image is the author's original work and was created using the BioRender application.

specialized equipment, such as the use of fluorescence microscopes to detect viral proteins, can limit their availability in some clinical settings, as described in **Figure 4** [27]. Furthermore, while fluorescence detection can identify protein or RNA viral, it may not distinguish between active and inactive infections, which can complicate clinical decision-making [23].

3. Molecular laboratories for polymerase chain reaction (PCR) diagnostic tests for respiratory infections

The molecular laboratory techniques for diagnosing respiratory infections have evolved significantly, with polymerase chain reaction (PCR) methods leading the way. This literature review will explore various PCR methodologies, including conventional PCR and reverse transcription PCR (RT-PCR), quantitative PCR, multiplex PCR, microarrays, and sequencing, highlighting their applications and advantages in the context of respiratory infections.

3.1 Conventional PCR and RT-PCR

Polymerase Chain Reaction (PCR) and reverse transcription PCR (RT-PCR) have revolutionized the field of diagnostics by providing rapid, sensitive, and specific detection of various pathogens. This literature review expounds on the mechanisms and applications of PCR in diagnostics, highlighting its advantages over traditional methods and its role in various medical contexts.

The conventional PCR process consists of three steps, which are related to the reaction temperature:

- Denaturation at 95°C
- Annealing between 55 and 70°C
- Extension at 72°C

The conventional reagents required for this reaction include a reaction buffer, magnesium ions, forward and reverse primers, Taq polymerase, and a DNA template. The PCR reaction takes place in a special tube containing a volume of 25 to 100 μL. Protocols typically involve 35–40 cycles of denaturation, annealing, and extension. After amplification, the resulting products are analyzed using agarose gels stained with intercalating dyes, allowing visualization under UV light as described in **Figure 5**.

PCR operates by amplifying specific DNA sequences, allowing for the detection of even minute quantities of genetic material. The technique was first conceptualized by Kary Mullis in 1983 and has since evolved into various forms, including real-time PCR and reverse-transcription PCR (RT-PCR) [28, 29]. Real-time PCR has gained prominence due to its ability to quantify DNA in real time, thus providing immediate results that are crucial in clinical settings [30, 31]. This method utilizes fluorescent dyes that emit signals proportional to the amount of amplified DNA, enhancing both sensitivity and specificity compared to conventional PCR methods [32].

The application of PCR in diagnosing infectious diseases is extensive. For instance, in the context of scrub typhus, studies have shown that nested PCR (N-PCR) is significantly more sensitive than conventional PCR (C-PCR), requiring only 200 pg. of DNA for detection compared to the 20 ng required by C-PCR [32]. This heightened sensitivity is critical for diagnosing infections caused by fastidious organisms that are difficult to culture, thereby facilitating timely treatment [32]. Similarly, PCR has been employed in the diagnosis of typhoid fever, where its sensitivity has been reported to be higher than that of traditional culture methods, establishing it as a valuable tool for detection [33].

In viral diagnostics, RT-PCR has become the preferred method for detecting RNA viruses, such as SARS-CoV-2. This technique has demonstrated superior sensitivity and specificity, making it a cornerstone of COVID-19 testing protocols [34, 35]. The ability of RT-PCR to detect viral RNA from various specimen types, including respiratory swabs, underscores its versatility and reliability in clinical diagnostics [34]. Moreover, PCR's utility extends beyond infectious diseases to include applications in oncology and genetic disorders. The technique has been pivotal in identifying mutations associated with various cancers, thereby aiding in personalized medicine approaches [30]. Additionally, PCR-based methods have been developed for the detection of genetic markers in hereditary diseases, enhancing diagnostic accuracy and enabling early intervention [36, 37].

Despite its numerous advantages, PCR is not without limitations. The presence of inhibitors in samples can affect the sensitivity of PCR assays, necessitating careful

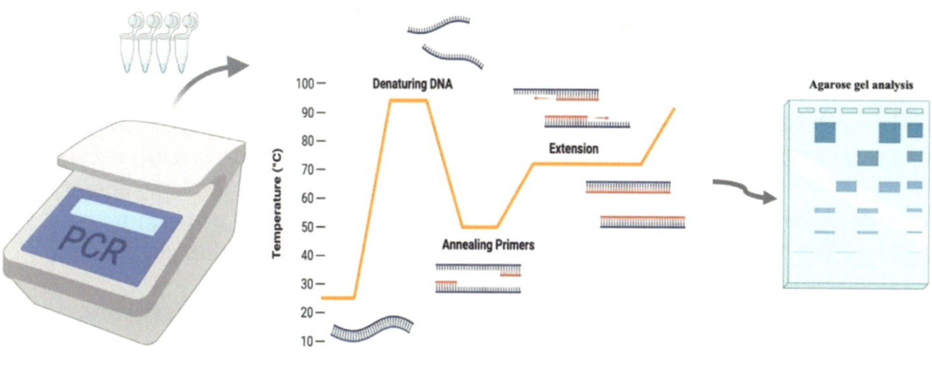

Figure 5.
Schematic diagram of conventional PCR protocol. Source: This image is the author's original work and was created using the BioRender application.

sample preparation and validation of extraction methods [31]. Furthermore, while PCR provides rapid results, the interpretation of these results requires skilled personnel to avoid misdiagnosis due to contamination or false positives [30, 31].

Conventional PCR has been a foundational technique in molecular diagnostics, allowing for the amplification of specific DNA sequences. However, its limitations include longer turnaround times and lower sensitivity compared to more advanced methods. RT-PCR, particularly in its quantitative form (qRT-PCR), has emerged as a powerful tool for detecting RNA viruses, such as influenza and respiratory syncytial virus (RSV), by converting RNA into complementary DNA (cDNA) before amplification. Studies have shown that RT-PCR provides rapid and sensitive detection of respiratory viruses, significantly improving diagnostic accuracy over traditional methods [38, 39]. For instance, Nakhaie et al. developed a multiplex RT-PCR that can simultaneously detect multiple viral pathogens, demonstrating the method's efficiency in clinical settings [40].

3.2 Real-time PCR and multiplex real-time PCR

Polymerase Chain Reaction (PCR) has evolved significantly since its inception, leading to the development of various methodologies, including quantitative PCR (qPCR) and multiplex PCR. This literature review aims to synthesize current research findings on these techniques, highlighting their applications, advantages, and comparative effectiveness.

Real-time PCR, also known as quantitative PCR, has emerged as a gold standard in molecular diagnostics due to its ability to provide quantitative data on nucleic acid concentrations in real time. It eliminates the need for post-amplification processing as described in **Figure 6**, which is a significant advantage over conventional PCR methods. For instance, Ramamurthy et al. demonstrated that real-time PCR not only saves time but also reduces the risk of cross-contamination compared to nested PCR techniques [41]. Similarly, Tozaki et al. noted that while real-time PCR is effective for quantifying low levels of viral RNA, the presence of PCR inhibitors in clinical samples can affect sensitivity [42]. Furthermore, the robustness of real-time PCR has been validated in various contexts, such as the detection of pathogens in human and veterinary medicine [43].

Multiplex PCR, which allows for the simultaneous amplification of multiple targets in a single reaction, has gained traction for its efficiency and cost-effectiveness. This technique is particularly useful in clinical diagnostics, where multiple pathogens need to be identified from a single sample. For example, Han et al. developed a duplex real-time PCR assay that successfully detected two viruses simultaneously, showcasing the method's high specificity and sensitivity as described in **Figure** 7 [44]. Additionally, Walochnik et al. reported the establishment of multiplex PCR protocols for the detection of Acanthamoeba, which demonstrated superior sensitivity and rapid results compared to traditional culture methods [45]. The ability to detect multiple targets in a single assay not only conserves reagents but also minimizes the time required for diagnosis, making multiplex PCR a valuable tool in clinical and research settings.

Multiplex PCR has revolutionized the diagnosis of respiratory infections by enabling the simultaneous detection of multiple pathogens in a single assay. This is particularly beneficial given the overlapping clinical presentations of respiratory viruses. Studies have demonstrated that multiplex PCR can detect a wide range of viral and bacterial pathogens, significantly improving diagnostic yield compared

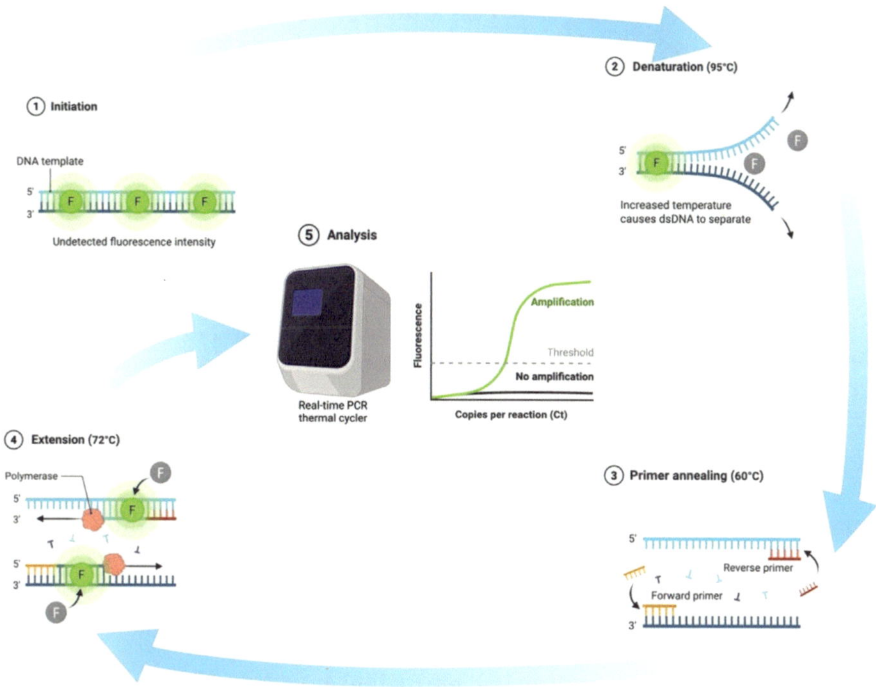

Figure 6.
Schematic diagram of real-time PCR. Source: This image is the author's original work and was created using the BioRender application.

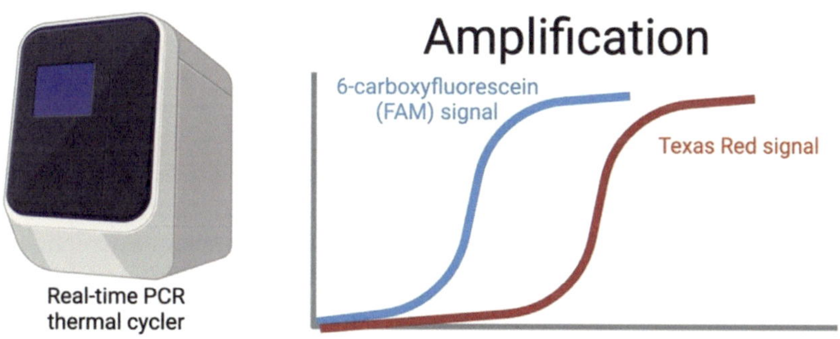

Figure 7.
Scheme of multiplex qPCR. Source: This image is the author's original work and was created using the BioRender application.

to conventional methods [46, 47]. For instance, Huang et al. reported that multiplex PCR assays are essential for identifying etiological agents in acute respiratory infections (ARIs), thus facilitating appropriate therapeutic interventions [48]. Furthermore, the ability to detect co-infections is critical, as many patients present with multiple pathogens, complicating treatment strategies [49].

The sensitivity and specificity of real-time PCR and multiplex PCR have been extensively documented. Cheng et al. found that real-time PCR exhibited higher sensitivity than nested PCR for detecting Plasmodium vivax, a significant finding in the context of malaria diagnostics [50]. Similarly, Ganguli et al. established that their duplex SYBR Green I-based real-time PCR assay offered higher detection rates than traditional PCR methods, further supporting the advantages of real-time approaches in clinical diagnostics. Moreover, studies have shown that real-time PCR can be up to 100 times more sensitive than conventional PCR, which is critical for early detection of infections [51].

Quantitative PCR enhances the capabilities of traditional PCR by allowing for the quantification of nucleic acids, which is crucial for understanding the viral load in patients. This method has been particularly useful in monitoring infections and guiding treatment decisions. The sensitivity of qPCR enables the detection of low viral loads, which is essential for early diagnosis and management of respiratory infections [2, 52]. For example, Lee et al. highlighted the importance of rapid molecular tests, including qPCR, in the timely identification of respiratory pathogens, which is critical for effective patient management [53].

3.3 Development of quantitative PCR innovations for SARS-CoV-2 and influenza A

Innovations in quantitative PCR, particularly droplet digital PCR (ddPCR) and advanced multiplex assays, have significantly enhanced the early and accurate detection of SARS-CoV-2. Traditional RT-PCR methods often yield false negatives, especially in cases with low viral loads, complicating timely diagnosis and transmission control [54, 55].

In contrast, ddPCR shows approximately tenfold greater sensitivity than RT-PCR, allowing for reliable detection even in low viral load samples. This improvement enhances diagnostic accuracy from 40 to 94% [55]. Additionally, the introduction of real-time fourplex TaqMan assays facilitates the simultaneous detection of multiple viral targets, including variants, with high specificity and sensitivity, detecting as few as 14 copies per reaction [56]. Furthermore, rapid diagnostic methods utilizing saliva samples have been optimized to enhance detection capabilities, making testing more accessible and efficient [57]. Collectively, these advancements enable the early identification of infected individuals, which is crucial for effective public health responses.

Recent innovations in quantitative PCR have significantly enhanced the sensitivity and speed of influenza A testing, addressing critical public health needs. The introduction of multiplex assays, such as the ProFast test, has improved sensitivity for subtyping influenza A viruses, allowing for the simultaneous detection of multiple subtypes—an essential factor for timely antiviral treatment decisions [58]. Additionally, droplet microfluidic technology has enabled the execution of up to eight parallel qPCR reactions, yielding results in just 35–40 minutes and detecting as few as 10 RNA copies per reaction, thus accelerating the diagnostic process [59]. Furthermore, long-range RT-qPCR assays have been developed to rapidly assess viral infectivity, correlating well with traditional methods while offering quicker results [60]. Collectively, these advances enhance influenza A diagnostic capabilities, facilitating improved surveillance and response strategies during outbreaks [61].

3.4 Microarray technology

Microarray technology complements PCR methods by allowing for the simultaneous analysis of thousands of nucleic acid sequences. This high-throughput approach is particularly useful for identifying a broad spectrum of respiratory pathogens, including those that are less common or newly emerging. Renois et al. utilized RT-PCR DNA microarray systems to detect various respiratory viruses, highlighting the method's ability to provide comprehensive diagnostic information [62]. The integration of microarrays with PCR techniques enhances the sensitivity and specificity of respiratory infection diagnostics, making it a valuable tool in clinical laboratories, as described in **Figure 8**.

3.4.1 Innovations in microarray technology for respiratory viruses

Innovations in microarray technology have significantly enhanced the early and accurate detection of respiratory viruses, which is essential for effective clinical management and public health responses. The development of comprehensive microarray systems allows for the simultaneous detection and subtyping of multiple respiratory viruses, including various influenza strains and newly identified pathogens, thereby improving diagnostic accuracy and speed [63, 64].

For instance, studies have demonstrated that multiplex RT-PCR DNA microarray systems can identify a wide range of respiratory viruses in clinical specimens, achieving high sensitivity and specificity compared to traditional methods [62, 65]. These advancements facilitate timely interventions, reduce reliance on antibiotics, and support the monitoring of viral outbreaks, ultimately contributing to improved patient outcomes and public health safety [64]. The integration of microarray technology into clinical virology practices represents a transformative step in the effective management of respiratory infections [65].

3.5 Next-generation sequencing (NGS) technologies in diagnosis

Next-generation sequencing technologies have emerged as a transformative tool in the diagnosis of infectious diseases, offering enhanced sensitivity and specificity compared to traditional methods, as described in **Figure 9**. The application of NGS in clinical settings has been particularly beneficial for identifying pathogens in complex cases where conventional culture methods may fail. For instance, Srichawla highlights the utility of plasma microbial cell-free DNA (cf-DNA) NGS in diagnosing intracranial abscesses, successfully identifying infections caused by *Fusobacterium nucleatum* and *Rothia mucilaginosa*, which underscores NGS's capability to detect multiple pathogens simultaneously [66]. Similarly, Liu's case report demonstrates that

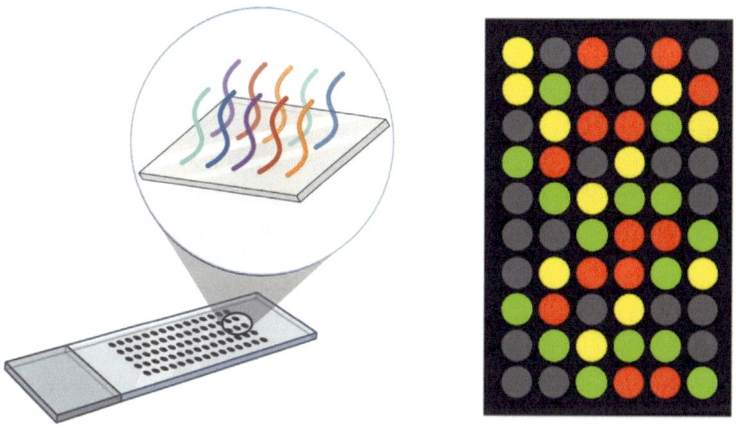

Figure 8.
Scheme of microarray technology. Source: This image is the author's original work and was created using the BioRender application.

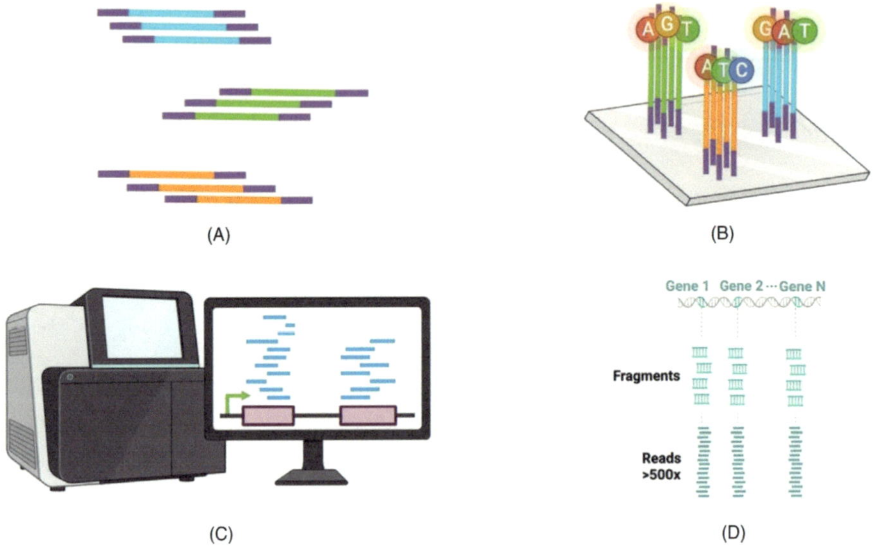

Figure 9.
Schematic diagram of next-generation sequencing. (A) Library preparation (B) Cluster amplification and sequencing (C) Alignment (D) Data analysis. Source: This image is the author's original work and was created using the BioRender application.

bronchoalveolar lavage fluid (BALF) NGS significantly improves the detection rates of bacteria in pulmonary infections, particularly in patients with rare pathogens and those who are immunocompromised [67].

The evolution of NGS technologies has facilitated their integration into clinical practice, particularly for diagnosing infections that are culture-negative or present atypical clinical features. For instance, Yin et al. discuss how NGS has revolutionized the diagnosis of periprosthetic joint infections by enabling the identification of uncommon pathogens that traditional methods might overlook [68]. This is echoed by Xing et al., who note that advancements in sequencing chemistries and computational capabilities have made NGS a valuable tool for rapid diagnosis in cases of fever without localizing features, as well as for culture-negative infections [69]. The ability of NGS to provide rapid and accurate diagnoses is further illustrated in the context of *Mycobacterium marinum* infections, where timely identification can significantly impact patient management [70].

Moreover, NGS has shown promise in diagnosing a wide range of infections, including those caused by fungi and atypical bacteria. For example, Zhang et al.'s report on the successful application of NGS to diagnose *Listeria monocytogenes* meningitis, highlighting its effectiveness in cases where traditional methods may be inadequate [71]. The potential of NGS to detect pathogens in challenging cases is further supported by studies on its use in diagnosing Q fever and other infections, where conventional diagnostic methods often fall short [69, 72].

The advantages of NGS extend beyond mere pathogen identification; they also include the ability to guide targeted antibiotic therapy. Kullar et al. emphasize that NGS can provide critical information about the infective organisms in culture-negative orthopedic infections, thereby facilitating more effective treatment strategies [73]. This is particularly important in the context of rising antibiotic resistance, where precise identification of pathogens can lead to better clinical outcomes.

Next-generation sequencing represents the forefront of molecular diagnostics, offering unparalleled depth of analysis for respiratory pathogens. This technique allows for the identification of known and novel viruses, providing insights into viral evolution and epidemiology. The application of NGS in respiratory infections has been shown to improve the understanding of viral diversity and the emergence of new strains, which is crucial for public health responses [74]. Additionally, sequencing can aid in the detection of co-infections and the characterization of pathogen resistance, further informing treatment decisions [75, 76].

3.5.1 Development of next-generation sequencing innovations for SARS-CoV-2 and influenza A

Recent innovations in next-generation sequencing have significantly enhanced the sensitivity and speed of SARS-CoV-2 testing, addressing the urgent need for effective diagnostic methods during the pandemic. Techniques such as SwabSeq allow for the pooling and barcoding of nasal and saliva samples, enabling the simultaneous testing of thousands of samples with a turnaround time of less than 24 hours while maintaining analytical sensitivity and specificity comparable to traditional qPCR tests [77]. Furthermore, the integration of CRISPR technology into NGS workflows has improved detection sensitivity for low-copy-number pathogens, making it possible to identify SARS-CoV-2 with accuracy similar to RT-qPCR while also allowing for variant strain typing and co-infection detection [78]. Collectively, these advancements not only streamline testing processes but also enhance the overall capacity for pandemic response [78, 79].

Similarly, NGS has transformed influenza A testing by enabling deep sequencing, which provides a comprehensive characterization of viral populations and identifies variants without the need for prior sequence knowledge [80]. The adaptation of the Illumina COVIDSeq™ Assay for influenza A and B sequencing has simplified workflows, achieving over 90% genomic coverage even at low viral loads—a critical factor for timely diagnostics [81]. Moreover, a "one-size-fits-all" NGS approach has demonstrated remarkable sensitivity, successfully identifying 99.4% of influenza-positive specimens. This method also uncovers essential genetic information for monitoring virulence and drug resistance [82]. These innovations not only expedite the identification of emerging strains but also enhance genomic surveillance, supporting more effective public health responses [83, 84].

4. Diagnosis using MXene-based biosensors

The utilization of MXenes in biosensing applications, particularly for the diagnosis of infections, has garnered significant attention due to their unique properties and versatile functionalities. MXenes, a class of two-dimensional materials, exhibit exceptional electrical conductivity, large surface area, and hydrophilicity, making them ideal candidates for biosensor development. This literature review synthesizes recent advancements in MXene-based biosensors, focusing on their application in infection diagnostics.

MXenes, particularly titanium carbide (Ti_3C_2), have demonstrated remarkable electrochemical properties that enhance the performance of biosensors, as described in **Figure 10**. For instance, Chia et al. reported a glucose biosensor based on pristine MXene that outperformed many existing technologies without the need for additional pretreatment with nanoparticles, highlighting the intrinsic advantages of MXenes in facilitating electron transfer processes [85]. This finding is corroborated by the work of Singh et al., who developed a functionalized Ti_3C_2 nanosheet biosensor for the point-of-care detection

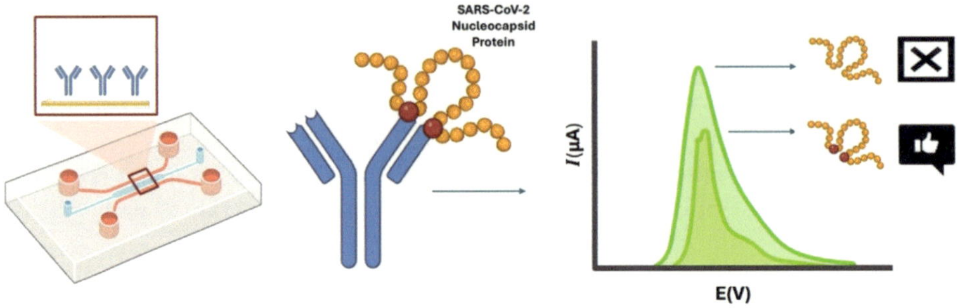

Figure 10.
Scheme of biosensor technology in detecting viral biomarkers. Source: This image is the author's original work and was created using the BioRender application.

of SARS-CoV-2 antigens, demonstrating the material's high sensitivity and specificity in detecting viral biomarkers [86]. The high specific surface area and excellent conductivity of MXenes contribute significantly to their effectiveness in electrochemical sensing applications, as noted by Yao et al., who emphasized the role of MXenes in various biosensing modalities, including enzyme-based and nucleic acid-based sensors [87].

The antimicrobial properties of MXenes further enhance their potential for infection control. Naser highlighted the diverse antimicrobial mechanisms of MXenes, which include membrane disruption and oxidative stress induction, making them effective against a range of pathogens, including bacteria, viruses, and fungi [88]. This broad-spectrum antimicrobial potential positions MXenes not only as diagnostic tools but also as therapeutic agents in infection management. Furthermore, the integration of MXenes into hydrogel matrices has been explored for their application in wound healing and drug delivery, showcasing their versatility in biomedical applications [89].

Recent innovations have also focused on hybrid biosensor designs that combine MXenes with other materials to improve detection capabilities. For example, Li et al. developed an MXene-graphene hybrid biosensor that utilizes nucleic acid probes for the advanced detection of SARS-CoV-2 and its variants, achieving high sensitivity and specificity [90]. The combination of MXenes with other nanomaterials, such as gold nanoparticles, has been shown to enhance the electrochemical performance of biosensors, as demonstrated by Liu et al., who reported superior electrochemical characteristics in their MXene-AuNPs hybrid platform [91].

Moreover, the application of surface-enhanced Raman scattering (SERS) technology in conjunction with MXenes has opened new avenues for sensitive virus detection. Peng et al. demonstrated that MXenes could significantly enhance SERS sensitivity for detecting SARS-CoV-2 proteins, providing a nondestructive and rapid detection method [92]. This capability is particularly crucial in clinical settings where timely diagnosis is essential for effective treatment.

In conclusion of the chapter, the diagnosis of respiratory diseases has seen significant advances thanks to the evolution of traditional techniques and the incorporation of innovative molecular technologies and biosensors. Traditional methods, such as viral culture and ELISA, have been essential for the identification of respiratory pathogens, although they have limitations in terms of time and sensitivity. However, recent innovations in ELISA and immunochromatographic tests have improved their efficiency, especially in the detection of viruses such as SARS-CoV-2 and influenza A.

On the other hand, molecular techniques, such as real-time PCR, multiplex PCR, and next-generation sequencing, have revolutionized diagnosis by offering greater sensitivity, specificity, and speed. These technologies allow for the simultaneous detection of multiple pathogens, the quantification of viral loads, and the identification of variants, which is crucial for clinical management and epidemiological surveillance.

Furthermore, MXenes-based biosensors have emerged as a promising tool, thanks to their electrochemical and antimicrobial properties. Its ability to integrate with other nanomaterials and technologies, such as surface-enhanced Raman scattering (SERS), has expanded its applicability in the rapid and accurate diagnosis of respiratory infections.

Together, these advances represent a comprehensive approach to the diagnosis of respiratory diseases, combining traditional methods with cutting-edge technologies. The choice of the appropriate technique should be based on clinical needs, resource availability, and the urgency of the diagnosis, thus ensuring effective and timely management of these infections, which significantly contributes to public health.

Acknowledgements

We deeply thank the University of Biological Sciences of the Universidad Autónoma de Nuevo León for their support in writing this book chapter.

Conflict of interest

The authors declare no conflict of interest.

Author details

Santiago Saavedra-Alonso[1,2]*, Ana Karina Chávez-Escamilla[1], Brenda Leticia Escobedo-Guajardo[3], Genoveva Alvarez-Ojeda[4], Carlos Alberto González-Villarreal[2], María Guadalupe Moreno-Treviño[2] and Juan Francisco Lugo-Ibarra[2]

1 Universidad Autónoma de Nuevo León, San Nicolás de los Garza Nuevo León, México

2 Universidad de Monterrey UDEM, Vicerrectoria de Ciencias de la Salud, San Pedro Garza García, Nuevo Léon, México

3 Centro de Investigación Biomédica del Noreste-IMSS, Monterrey, Nuevo León, México

4 INIFAP-Campo Experimental Río Bravo, Tamaulipas, México

*Address all correspondence to: ssaavedraln@uanl.edu.mx

References

[1] Kawase M, Suwa R, Sugimoto S, Kakizaki M, Kume Y, Chishiki M, et al. Evidence of the simultaneous replications of active viruses in specimens positive for multiple respiratory viruses. Microbiology Spectrum. 2024;**12**(1):e0192023

[2] Olofsson S, Brittain-Long R, Andersson LM, Westin J, Lindh M. PCR for detection of respiratory viruses: Seasonal variations of virus infections. Expert Review of Anti-Infective Therapy. 2011;**9**(8):615-626

[3] Calderaro A, Arcangeletti MC, Rodighiero I, Buttrini M, Montecchini S, Vasile Simone R, et al. Identification of different respiratory viruses, after a cell culture step, by matrix assisted laser desorption/ionization time of flight mass spectrometry (MALDI-TOF MS). Scientific Reports. 2016;**6**:36082

[4] Sattler T, Wodak E, Revilla-Fernández S, Schmoll F. Comparison of different commercial ELISAs for detection of antibodies against porcine respiratory and reproductive syndrome virus in serum. BMC Veterinary Research. 2014;**10**:300

[5] Rissin DM, Kan CW, Campbell TG, Howes SC, Fournier DR, Song L, et al. Single-molecule enzyme-linked immunosorbent assay detects serum proteins at subfemtomolar concentrations. Nature Biotechnology. 2010;**28**(6):595-599

[6] Xu L, Zhang Z, Zhang Q, Zhang W, Yu L, Wang D, et al. An on-site simultaneous semi-quantification of Aflatoxin B1, zearalenone, and T-2 toxin in maize- and cereal-based feed via multicolor immunochromatographic assay. Toxins (Basel). 2018;**10**(2)

[7] Zedan HT, Yassine HM, Al-Sadeq DW, Liu N, Qotba H, Nicolai E, et al. Evaluation of commercially available fully automated and ELISA-based assays for detecting anti-SARS-CoV-2 neutralizing antibodies. Scientific Reports. 2022;**12**(1):19020

[8] Schöler L, Le-Trilling VTK, Eilbrecht M, Mennerich D, Anastasiou OE, Krawczyk A, et al. A novel In-cell ELISA assay allows rapid and automated quantification of SARS-CoV-2 to analyze neutralizing antibodies and antiviral compounds. Frontiers in Immunology. 2020;**11**:573526

[9] Perkmann T, Koller T, Perkmann-Nagele N, Ozsvar-Kozma M, Eyre D, Matthews P, et al. Increasing test specificity without impairing sensitivity: Lessons learned from SARS-CoV-2 serology. Journal of Clinical Pathology. 2023;**76**(11):770-777

[10] Mehdi F, Chattopadhyay S, Thiruvengadam R, Yadav S, Kumar M, Sinha SK, et al. Development of a fast SARS-CoV-2 IgG ELISA, based on receptor-binding domain, and its comparative evaluation using temporally segregated samples from RT-PCR positive individuals. Frontiers in Microbiology. 2020;**11**:618097

[11] Ahmed SR, Kim J, Suzuki T, Lee J, Park EY. Detection of influenza virus using peroxidase-mimic of gold nanoparticles. Biotechnology and Bioengineering. 2016;**113**(10):2298-2303

[12] Casini D, Fontani P, Ruggiero P, Balducci E, Berti D. A rapid ELISA method to improve the automated test throughput. Journal of Analytical & Bioanalytical Techniques. 2015;**6**(13):1-4

[13] Bamrungsap S, Apiwat C, Chantima W, Dharakul T, Wiriyachaiporn N. Rapid and sensitive lateral flow immunoassay for influenza antigen using fluorescently-doped silica nanoparticles. Microchimica Acta. 2014;**181**(1):223-230

[14] Selim HS, Hashish MH. Performance of a rapid test versus real-time PCR for diagnosis of H1N1 swine flu. The Journal of the Egyptian Public Health Association. 2014;**89**(2):96-99

[15] Wang W, Liu L, Xu L, Kuang H, Zhu J, Xu C. Gold-nanoparticle-based multiplexed immunochromatographic strip for simultaneous detection of staphylococcal enterotoxin A, B, C, D, and E. Particle & Particle Systems Characterization. 2016;**33**(7):388-395

[16] Zeng N, Wang Z, Zineddin B, Li Y, Du M, Xiao L, et al. Image-based quantitative analysis of gold immunochromatographic strip via cellular neural network approach. IEEE Transactions on Medical Imaging. 2014;**33**(5):1129-1136

[17] Gantelius J, Bass T, Sjöberg R, Nilsson P, Andersson-Svahn H. A lateral flow protein microarray for rapid and sensitive antibody assays. International Journal of Molecular Sciences. 2011;**12**(11):7748-7759

[18] Sotnikov DV, Safenkova IV, Zherdev AV, Avdienko VG, Kozlova IV, Babayan SS, et al. A mechanism of gold nanoparticle aggregation by immunoglobulin G preparation. Applied Sciences [Internet]. 2020;**10**(2)

[19] Zhang J, Xia Y-K, Chen M, Wu D-Z, Cai S-X, Liu M-M, et al. A fluorescent aptasensor based on DNA-scaffolded silver nanoclusters coupling with Zn(II)-ion signal-enhancement for simultaneous detection of OTA and AFB1. Sensors and Actuators B: Chemical. 2016;**235**:79-85

[20] Maragos CM. Multiplexed biosensors for mycotoxins. Journal of AOAC International. 2016;**99**(4):849-860

[21] Lv G, Shi L, Liu Y, Sun X, Mu K. Epidemiological characteristics of common respiratory pathogens in children. Scientific Reports. 2024;**14**(1):16299

[22] Nabeya D, Kinjo T, Ueno S, Setoguchi M, Nishiyama N, Kami W, et al. Characteristics of patients with viral infections of the lower respiratory tract: A retrospective study. Medicine (Baltimore). 2022;**101**(38):e30819

[23] Pagliano P, Sellitto C, Conti V, Ascione T, Esposito S. Characteristics of viral pneumonia in the COVID-19 era: An update. Infection. 2021;**49**(4):607-616

[24] Rashida Akter K, Md Nazrul I, Shahina T, Ahmed S, Md Abdullah Y. Validity of immunofluorescence test for the detection of respiratory viruses causing acute lower respiratory tract infection among under five children. International Journal of Microbiology and Biotechnology. 2018;**3**(1):7-10

[25] Brittain-Long R, Westin J, Olofsson S, Lindh M, Andersson LM. Access to a polymerase chain reaction assay method targeting 13 respiratory viruses can reduce antibiotics: A randomised, controlled trial. BMC Medicine. 2011;**9**:44

[26] Avolio M, Venturini S, De Rosa R, Crapis M, Basaglia G. Epidemiology of respiratory virus before and during COVID-19 pandemic. Le Infezioni in Medicina. 2022;**30**(1):104-108

[27] Balada-Llasat JM, LaRue H, Kelly C, Rigali L, Pancholi P. Evaluation of commercial ResPlex II v2.0, MultiCode-PLx, and xTAG respiratory viral panels for the diagnosis of respiratory viral

infections in adults. Journal of Clinical Virology. 2011;**50**(1):42-45

[28] Chang CC, Chen CC, Wei SC, Lu HH, Liang YH, Lin CW. Diagnostic devices for isothermal nucleic acid amplification. Sensors (Basel). 2012;**12**(6):8319-8337

[29] Fukui K, Bessho Y, Shimada A, Yokoyama S, Kuramitsu S. Thermostable mismatch-recognizing protein MutS suppresses nonspecific amplification during polymerase chain reaction (PCR). International Journal of Molecular Sciences. 2013;**14**(3):6436-6453

[30] Schrick L, Nitsche A. Pitfalls in PCR troubleshooting: Expect the unexpected? Biomolecular Detection and Quantification. 2016;**6**:1-3

[31] Abdel-Hamid NH, Beleta EIM, Kelany MA, Ismail RI, Shalaby NA, Khafagi MHM. Validation of real-time polymerase chain reaction versus conventional polymerase chain reaction for diagnosis of brucellosis in cattle sera. Vet World. 2021;**14**(1):144-154

[32] Kim GH, Kim MJ, Choi HJ, Koo MJ, Kim MJ, Min JG, et al. Evaluation of a novel TaqMan probe-based real-time polymerase chain reaction (PCR) assay for detection and quantitation of red sea bream iridovirus. Fisheries and Aquatic Sciences. 2021;**24**(11):351-359

[33] Das S, Ray U, Akhter I, Chattopadhyay A, Paul DK, Dutta S. Evaluation of fliC-d based direct blood PCR assays for typhoid diagnosis. BMC Microbiology. 2016;**16**(1):108

[34] Imborek KL, Krasowski MD, Natvig P, Merrill AE, Diekema DJ, Ford BA. Experience with Pretravel testing for SARS-CoV-2 at an Academic Medical Center. Academic Pathology. 2021;**8**:23742895211010247

[35] Symons R, Beath K, Dangis A, Lefever S, Smismans A, De Bruecker Y, et al. A statistical framework to estimate diagnostic test performance for COVID-19. Clinical Radiology. 2021;**76**(1):75.e1-75.e3

[36] Jha H, Baveja CP, Kamal V, Agarwal PN, Saxena S, Dhakad MS, et al. Comparative diagnostic of cervical tuberculous lymphadenitis: PCR is a fast, efficient, and improved diagnostic approach. Canadian Journal of Infectious Diseases and Medical Microbiology. 2023;**2023**:3312250

[37] Roberts T, Barratt J, Harkness J, Ellis J, Stark D. Comparison of microscopy, culture, and conventional polymerase chain reaction for detection of *Blastocystis* sp. in clinical stool samples. The American Journal of Tropical Medicine and Hygiene. 2011;**84**(2):308-312

[38] Martins Júnior RB, Carney S, Goldemberg D, Bonine L, Spano LC, Siqueira M, et al. Detection of respiratory viruses by real-time polymerase chain reaction in outpatients with acute respiratory infection. Memórias do Instituto Oswaldo Cruz. 2014;**109**(6):716-721

[39] Neopane P, Nypaver J, Shrestha R, Beqaj S. Performance evaluation of TaqMan SARS-CoV-2, flu A/B, RSV RT-PCR multiplex assay for the detection of respiratory viruses. Infection and Drug Resistance. 2022;**15**:5411-5423

[40] Nakhaie M, Soleimanjahi H, Mollaie HR, Arabzadeh SMA. Development of multiplex reverse transcription-polymerase chain reaction for simultaneous detection of influenza A, B and adenoviruses. Iranian Journal of Pathology. 2018;**13**(1):54-62

[41] Ramamurthy M, Alexander M, Aaron S, Kannangai R, Ravi V,

Sridharan G, et al. Comparison of a conventional polymerase chain reaction with real-time polymerase chain reaction for the detection of neurotropic viruses in cerebrospinal fluid samples. Indian Journal of Medical Microbiology. 2011;**29**(2):102-109

[42] Tozaki T, Ohnuma A, Iwai S, Kikuchi M, Ishige T, Kakoi H, et al. Robustness of digital PCR and real-time PCR in transgene detection for gene-doping control. Analytical Chemistry. 2021;**93**(18):7133-7139

[43] Wan C, Chen C, Cheng L, Chen H, Fu Q, Shi S, et al. Specific detection of Muscovy duck parvovirus infection by TaqMan-based real-time PCR assay. BMC Veterinary Research. 2018;**14**(1):267

[44] Han HY, Zheng HH, Zhao Y, Tian RB, Xu PL, Hou HL, et al. Development of a SYBR green I-based duplex real-time fluorescence quantitative PCR assay for the simultaneous detection of porcine epidemic diarrhea virus and porcine circovirus 3. Molecular and Cellular Probes. 2019;**44**:44-50

[45] Walochnik J, Scheikl U, Haller-Schober EM. Twenty years of acanthamoeba diagnostics in Austria. The Journal of Eukaryotic Microbiology. 2015;**62**(1):3-11

[46] Sollip K, Ki-Won E, Chong-Rae C, Um TH. Comparison of the ability of multiplex and Singleplex PCR to detect human respiratory viruses. Laboratory Medicine Online. 2016;**6**(4):240-245

[47] Saarela E, Renko M, Uhari M, Pokka T, Kauma H, Ruuska TS. Multiplex PCR for respiratory bacteria in acute care. APMIS. 2024;**132**(6):444-451

[48] Huang HS, Tsai CL, Chang J, Hsu TC, Lin S, Lee CC. Multiplex PCR system for the rapid diagnosis of respiratory virus infection: Systematic review and meta-analysis. Clinical Microbiology and Infection. 2018;**24**(10):1055-1063

[49] Zhang G, Hu Y, Wang H, Zhang L, Bao Y, Zhou X. High incidence of multiple viral infections identified in upper respiratory tract infected children under three years of age in Shanghai, China. PLoS One. 2012;**7**(9):e44568

[50] Cheng J, Carter I, Wang L, Taylor P. Real-time PCR for laboratory diagnosis of Acanthamoeba keratitis. Microbiology Australia. 2011;**32**(2):111-112

[51] Arastehfar A, Fang W, Pan W, Liao W, Yan L, Boekhout T. Identification of nine cryptic species of *Candida albicans*, *C. Glabrata*, and *C. Parapsilosis* complexes using one-step multiplex PCR. BMC Infectious Diseases. 2018;**18**(1):480

[52] Baghdadi JD, O'Hara LM, Johnson JK, Krein SL, Harris AD, Morgan DJ. Diagnostic stewardship to support optimal use of multiplex molecular respiratory panels: A survey from the Society for Healthcare Epidemiology of America Research Network. Infection Control and Hospital Epidemiology. 2023;**44**(11):1823-1828

[53] Lee JM, Lee JH, Kim YK. Laboratory impact of rapid molecular tests used for the detection of respiratory pathogens. Clinical Laboratory. 2018;**64**(9):1545-1551

[54] Zhang J, Han J, Liang Y, Liu W, Wang X, Liao ZY, et al., editors. The Development of a Droplet Digital PCR for Accurate Detection of SARS-CoV-2 by Simultaneous Determination of Dual Gene Targets. 2022. Available from: https://europepmc.org/article/ppr/ppr566424

[55] Suo T, Liu X, Feng J, Guo M, Hu W, Guo D, et al. ddPCR: A more accurate tool for SARS-CoV-2 detection in low viral load specimens. Emerging Microbes & Infections. 2020;**9**(1):1259-1268

[56] Durand M, Thibault P, Lévesque S, Brault A, Carignan A, Valiquette L, et al. Detection of severe acute respiratory syndrome coronavirus 2 (SARS-CoV-2) and its first variants in fourplex real-time quantitative reverse transcription-PCR assays. Microbial Cell (Graz, Austria). 2022;**9**(1):1-20

[57] Tokuyama-Toda R, Terada-Ito C, Muraoka M, Horiuchi T, Amemiya T, Fukuoka A, et al. Improving the detection sensitivity of a new rapid diagnostic technology for severe acute respiratory syndrome coronavirus 2 using a trace amount of saliva. Diagnostics (Basel). 2022;**12**(11)

[58] Mosammaparast N, Rossi RF, Smole S, McAdam AJ. Improved sensitivity of a commercial reverse transcription-PCR test for subtyping of the 2009 H1N1 influenza A virus. Journal of Clinical Microbiology. 2011;**49**(3):1188

[59] Prakash R, Pabbaraju K, Wong S, Wong A, Tellier R, Kaler KVIS. Multiplex, quantitative, reverse transcription PCR detection of influenza viruses using droplet microfluidic technology. Micromachines [Internet]. 2015;**6**(1):63-79

[60] Nakaya Y, Fukuda T, Ashiba H, Yasuura M, Fujimaki M. Quick assessment of influenza A virus infectivity with a long-range reverse-transcription quantitative polymerase chain reaction assay. BMC Infectious Diseases. 2020;**20**(1):585

[61] Szewczuk E, Thapa K, Anninos T, McPhie K, Higgins G, Dwyer DE, et al. Rapid semi-automated quantitative multiplex tandem PCR (MT-PCR) assays for the differential diagnosis of influenza-like illness. BMC Infectious Diseases. 2010;**10**:113

[62] Renois F, Talmud D, Huguenin A, Moutte L, Strady C, Cousson J, et al. Rapid detection of respiratory tract viral infections and coinfections in patients with influenza-like illnesses by use of reverse transcription-PCR DNA microarray systems. Journal of Clinical Microbiology. 2010;**48**(11):3836-3842

[63] Quan PL, Palacios G, Jabado OJ, Conlan S, Hirschberg DL, Pozo F, et al. Detection of respiratory viruses and subtype identification of influenza A viruses by GreeneChipResp oligonucleotide microarray. Journal of Clinical Microbiology. 2007;**45**(8):2359-2364

[64] Zhang N, Wang L, Deng X, Liang R, Su M, He C, et al. Recent advances in the detection of respiratory virus infection in humans. Journal of Medical Virology. 2020;**92**(4):408-417

[65] Huguenin A, Moutte L, Renois F, Leveque N, Talmud D, Abely M, et al. Broad respiratory virus detection in infants hospitalized for bronchiolitis by use of a multiplex RT-PCR DNA microarray system. Journal of Medical Virology. 2012;**84**(6):979-985

[66] Srichawla BS. Plasma microbial cell-free DNA (CF-DNA) next-generation sequencing in diagnosing intracranial abscesses: Pathophysiology and a scoping review of the literature. Cureus. 2022;**14**(8):e28172

[67] Liu Y, Li Z, Fu H, Ruan W, Wang H, Ding Y, et al. The first case report: Diagnosis and management of necrotizing *Fusobacterium* lung abscess via BALF next-generation

sequencing. BMC Infectious Diseases. 2024;**24**(1):218

[68] Yin H, Xu D, Wang D. Diagnostic value of next-generation sequencing to detect periprosthetic joint infection. BMC Musculoskeletal Disorders. 2021;**22**(1):252

[69] Xing F, Ye H, Deng C, Sun L, Yuan Y, Lu Q, et al. Diverse and atypical manifestations of Q fever in a metropolitan city hospital: Emerging role of next-generation sequencing for laboratory diagnosis of *Coxiella burnetii*. PLoS Neglected Tropical Diseases. 2022;**16**(4):e0010364

[70] Xing F, Lo SKF, Ma Y, Ip JD, Chan WM, Zhou M, et al. Rapid Diagnosis of Mycobacterium marinum Infection by Next-Generation Sequencing: A Case Report. Frontiers in Medicine (Lausanne). 2022;**9**:824122

[71] Xing F, Hung DLL, Lo SKF, Chen S, Lau SKP, Woo PCY. Next-generation sequencing-based diagnosis of *Bacteremic Listeria monocytogenes* meningitis in a patient with anti-interferon gamma: Autoantibodies: A case report. Infectious Microbes & Diseases. 2022;**4**(1)

[72] Xu A, Zhu H, Gao B, Weng H, Ding Z, Li M, et al. Diagnosis of severe community-acquired pneumonia caused by *Acinetobacter baumannii* through next-generation sequencing: A case report. BMC Infectious Diseases. 2020;**20**(1):45

[73] Kullar R, Chisari E, Snyder J, Cooper C, Parvizi J, Sniffen J. Next-generation sequencing supports targeted antibiotic treatment for culture negative orthopedic infections. Clinical Infectious Diseases. 2023;**76**(2):359-364

[74] Yuan G, Wang H, Zhao Y, Mao E, Li M, Wang R, et al. Early identification and severity prediction of acute respiratory infection (ESAR): A study protocol for a randomized controlled trial. BMC Infectious Diseases. 2022;**22**(1):632

[75] Alimi Y, Lim WS, Lansbury L, Leonardi-Bee J, Nguyen-Van-Tam JS. Systematic review of respiratory viral pathogens identified in adults with community-acquired pneumonia in Europe. Journal of Clinical Virology. 2017;**95**:26-35

[76] Li J, Tao Y, Tang M, Du B, Xia Y, Mo X, et al. Rapid detection of respiratory organisms with the Film Array respiratory panel in a large children's hospital in China. BMC Infectious Diseases. 2018;**18**(1):510

[77] Bloom JS, Sathe L, Munugala C, Jones EM, Gasperini M, Lubock NB, et al. Massively scaled-up testing for SARS-CoV-2 RNA via next-generation sequencing of pooled and barcoded nasal and saliva samples. Nature Biomedical Engineering. 2021;**5**(7):657-665

[78] Chan AP, Siddique A, Desplat Y, Choi Y, Ranganathan S, Choudhary KS, et al. A CRISPR-enhanced metagenomic NGS test to improve pandemic preparedness. Cell Reports Methods. 2023;**3**(5):100463

[79] Chiara M, D'Erchia AM, Gissi C, Manzari C, Parisi A, Resta N, et al. Next generation sequencing of SARS-CoV-2 genomes: Challenges, applications and opportunities. Briefings in Bioinformatics. 2021;**22**(2):616-630

[80] Lee DH. Complete genome sequencing of influenza A viruses using next-generation sequencing. Methods in Molecular Biology. 2020;**2123**:69-79

[81] Lin Y, Koble J, Prashar P, Pottekat A, Middle C, Kuersten S, et al. A Sequencing and Subtyping Protocol for Influenza

A and B Viruses Using Illumina® COVIDSeq™ Assay Kit. 2023. Available from: https://www.protocols.io/view/a-sequencing-and-subtyping-protocol-for-influenza-n2bvj8mrxgk5/v1 [Accessed: 1 November 2023]

[82] Zhao J, Liu J, Vemula SV, Lin C, Tan J, Ragupathy V, et al. Sensitive detection and simultaneous discrimination of influenza A and B viruses in nasopharyngeal swabs in a single assay using next-generation sequencing-based diagnostics. PLoS One. 2016;**11**(9):e0163175

[83] Ali R, Blackburn RM, Kozlakidis Z. Next-generation sequencing and influenza virus: A short review of the published implementation attempts. HAYATI Journal of Biosciences. 2016;**23**(4):155-159

[84] Laassri M, Plant EP, Zagorodnyaya T, Rodionova E, Voskanian-Kordi A, Simonyan V, et al. Application of the new generation of sequencing technologies for evaluation of genetic consistency of influenza A vaccine viruses. In: Baddour MM, editor. Steps Forwards in Diagnosing and Controlling Influenza. Rijeka: IntechOpen; 2016

[85] Chia HL, Mayorga-Martinez CC, Antonatos N, Sofer Z, Gonzalez-Julian JJ, Webster RD, et al. MXene titanium carbide-based biosensor: Strong dependence of exfoliation method on performance. Analytical Chemistry. 2020;**92**(3):2452-2459

[86] Singh C, Höfs S, Konthur Z, Hodoroaba V-D, Radnik J, Schenk JA, et al. Functionalized Ti3C2Tx nanosheets based biosensor for point-of-care detection of SARS-CoV-2 antigen. ACS Applied Engineering Materials. 2023;**1**(1):495-507

[87] Yao B, Yao J, Fan Z, Zhao J, Zhang K, Huang W. Rapid advances of versatile MXenes for electrochemical enzyme-based biosensors, immunosensors, and nucleic acid-based biosensors. ChemElectroChem. 2022;**9**(11):e202200103

[88] Habeeb Naser I, Ali Naeem Y, Ali E, Yarab Hamed A, Farhan Muften N, Turky Maan F, et al. Revolutionizing infection control: Harnessing MXene-based nanostructures for versatile antimicrobial strategies and healthcare advancements. Chemistry & Biodiversity. 2024;**21**(5):e202400366

[89] Hamzehlouy A, Tavakoli Dare M, Shahi F, Dawi EA, Khonakdar HA. Recent advances in potential biomedical applications of MXene-based hydrogels. Polymers for Advanced Technologies. 2024;**35**(12):e70008

[90] Li J, Zhang Y, Wei C, Li Y, Peng Z, Chuang H-Y, et al. Advanced detection of SARS-CoV-2 and omicron variants via MXene-graphene hybrid biosensors utilizing nucleic acid probes. ACS Applied Nano Materials. 2024;**7**(24):28255-28272

[91] Liu X, Qiu Y, Jiang D, Li F, Gan Y, Zhu Y, et al. Covalently grafting first-generation PAMAM dendrimers onto MXenes with self-adsorbed AuNPs for use as a functional nanoplatform for highly sensitive electrochemical biosensing of cTnT. Microsystems & Nanoengineering. 2022;**8**:35

[92] Peng Y, Lin C, Long L, Masaki T, Tang M, Yang L, et al. Charge-transfer resonance and electromagnetic enhancement synergistically enabling MXenes with excellent SERS sensitivity for SARS-CoV-2 S protein detection. Nano-micro Letters. 2021;**13**:52

Chapter 4

Perspective Chapter: Advancements in Cancer Biomarkers – Transforming Diagnostics and Therapeutic Strategies in Precision Oncology

Tatiana de Almeida Simão, Jennifer Vieira Gomes, Diego José Gomes de Paula and Suzana Pinheiro de Oliveira Ribeiro

Abstract

Cancer treatment has long been a complex challenge, but precision oncology has transformed the field by driving the development of targeted therapies and refining existing approaches. At the heart of this revolution are molecular biomarkers, essential tools for identifying patients who will benefit most from personalized treatments. Biomarkers have vast potential in oncology, aiding in risk assessment, screening, prognosis, diagnosis, treatment response prediction, and disease monitoring. Several biomarkers are already integral to clinical practice. For example, *BRCA1* and *BRCA2* gene variants are linked to higher risks of breast and ovarian cancers. In contrast, HER2 receptor amplification in breast cancer—the most common malignancy among women—guides treatment decisions due to its association with poorer outcomes. Beyond traditional markers, epigenetics and microbiome research advances have expanded the biomarker landscape. Epigenetic changes, such as *SEPT9* gene methylation, show promise for early colorectal cancer detection, while microbiome studies reveal its role in cancer development and innovative therapies. As biomarker research accelerates, it is critical to search for markers with greater sensitivity, specificity, and predictive power. These advancements improve diagnostic accuracy and therapeutic outcomes, ultimately enhancing cancer care and patient survival.

Keywords: precision oncology, molecular biomarkers, carcinogenesis, target therapies, prognostic biomarkers

1. Introduction

Cancer remains one of the leading causes of mortality worldwide, with an estimated 20 million new cases and 9.7 million cancer-related deaths reported in 2022 [1]. Projections indicate that by 2050, new cancer cases will reach 35 million, representing a staggering 77% increase compared to 2022 [2]. Early cancer detection and therapeutic efficacy remain significant challenges despite significant advancements in oncology that aim to improve patient outcomes.

Many types of malignant tumors are diagnosed at advanced stages, which leads to limited treatment options and reduced survival rates. In this context, tumor biomarkers have emerged as essential tools, advancing precision medicine by offering personalized diagnostic and therapeutic strategies [3].

According to the National Cancer Institute (NCI), a cancer biomarker is "a biological molecule found in blood, other body fluids, or tissues that signal a normal or abnormal process, condition, or disease. Biomarkers can also be used to assess treatment response and disease progression" [4]. The continuous evolution of molecular biology, genomics, and high-throughput technologies has improved biomarkers research, increasing their accuracy and applicability in oncology. However, despite significant progress, translating biomarkers from research to routine clinical practice remains challenging, requiring robust analytical performance, cost-effectiveness assessments, and massive validation [5].

1.1 Cancer biomarkers classification

Biomarkers have a fundamental role in oncology, offering a critical understanding of cancer detection, prognosis, and treatment response. Their classification is based on their clinical utility, contributing to a more precise and personalized approach to cancer management (**Figure 1**).

- Diagnostic biomarkers: These biomarkers facilitate early detection and distinguish malignant from benign conditions. Examples include Prostate-specific antigen (PSA) for prostate cancer and Alpha-fetoprotein (AFP) for hepatocellular carcinoma. However, these biomarkers are imperfect, as PSA levels can be elevated in benign prostatic conditions such as prostatitis and benign prostatic hyperplasia [6]. At the same time, AFP can also be increased in non-malignant liver diseases such as cirrhosis and hepatitis, leading to potential false positives and limitations in specificity [7].

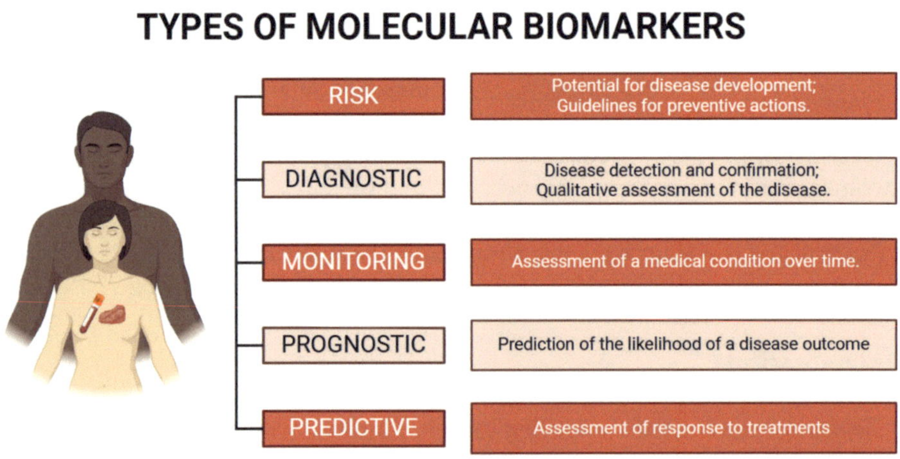

Figure 1.
Types of molecular biomarkers most commonly used in clinical and research settings.

- Prognostic biomarkers: Provide insights into disease progression and patient outcomes, independent of treatment. For example, human epidermal growth factor receptor type 2 (HER2) overexpression in breast cancer is associated with increased tumor proliferation, higher metastatic potential, and more há aggressive disease [8], often requiring targeted therapies such as trastuzumab (Herceptin) to improve patient outcomes. Similarly, *TP53* mutations, which disrupt the tumor suppressor function of the P53 protein, are frequently linked to genomic instability, resistance to therapy, and overall poorer prognosis in multiple cancer types, including lung, ovarian, and pancreatic cancer [9]. Understanding these biomarkers enables better risk assessment and helps guide treatment decisions, even when they do not directly influence therapeutic choices.

- Predictive biomarkers: Aid treatment selection by identifying patients more likely to respond to specific therapies. Epidermal growth factor receptor (*EGFR*) mutations serve as predictive biomarkers in non-small cell lung cancer (NSCLC), as they help identify patients who are likely to respond to tyrosine kinase inhibitors (TKIs) such as erlotinib, egfitinib, afatinib, and osimertinib. These mutations occur in the *EGFR* gene, leading to the overactivation of downstream signaling pathways that drive tumor growth and survival. Patients with activating *EGFR* mutations (such as exon 19 deletions and L858R substitution in exon 21) tend to respond well to TKIs, which block EGFR signaling, inhibiting tumor proliferation and promoting apoptosis. However, resistance mechanisms like the T790M mutation can develop over time, requiring next-generation TKIs like Osimertinib [10]. Similarly, PD-L1 expression serves as a predictive biomarker for the use of immune checkpoint inhibitors (ICIs), such as pembrolizumab, nivolumab, and atezolizumab, which target the PD-1/PD-L1 pathway. PD-L1 (programmed death-ligand 1) is a protein expressed on tumor cells that interacts with PD-1 (programmed death-1) on T cells, suppressing the immune response and allowing tumors to evade immune surveillance. High PD-L1 expression ($\geq$50% in some clinical guidelines) is associated with a greater likelihood of response to PD-1/PD-L1 inhibitors, as these therapies work by blocking the PD-1/PD-L1 interaction, thereby reinvigorating the immune system to attack cancer cells. However, not all patients with high PD-L1 expressions respond to ICIs, and additional biomarkers, such as tumor mutational burden (TMB) and microsatellite instability (MSI-H), are being explored to improve patient selection for immunotherapy [11].

- Monitoring biomarkers: Assess tumor burden, recurrence risk, and treatment efficacy. Carcinoembryonic antigen (CEA) is a widely used tumor-associated biomarker for monitoring colorectal cancer (CRC) progression. CEA is a glycoprotein involved in cell adhesion, and although it is typically produced during fetal development, its expression is minimal in healthy adults. However, elevated levels of CEA in the blood are frequently associated with colorectal cancer, as well as other malignancies such as gastric, pancreatic, and lung cancers. In clinical practice, CEA is not used for early cancer detection due to its limited specificity, as elevations can also occur in benign conditions such as inflammatory bowel disease, liver disease, and smoking. Instead, it is primarily used as a monitoring tool to track treatment response, disease recurrence, and metastatic progression in CRC patients. After surgical resection or chemotherapy, a declining CEA level suggests treatment success. In contrast, persistent or rising levels may indicate residual or recurrent disease, prompting further investigation with imaging and additional tests [12, 13]. In contrast, circulating tumor DNA (ctDNA) is an emerging, highly sensitive biomarker for minimal residual disease (MRD) detection. ctDNA consists of tumor-derived DNA fragments released into the bloodstream by apoptotic or necrotic cancer cells. Unlike CEA, which provides a general tumor burden indicator, ctDNA offers a more precise and dynamic assessment of residual cancer presence at the molecular level. Even when imaging scans appear clear after treatment, ctDNA can detect microscopic diseases that may lead to recurrence, making it a powerful tool for early relapse prediction. Studies have shown that patients with detectable ctDNA post-surgery have a significantly higher risk of recurrence, whereas those with undetectable ctDNA levels are more likely to remain in remission. Additionally, ctDNA can provide insights into tumor evolution and treatment resistance, allowing for personalized therapeutic adjustments based on real-time molecular profiling. While CEA remains a standard biomarker for colorectal cancer monitoring, ctDNA is revolutionizing post-treatment surveillance, enabling earlier intervention in patients with MRD and improving long-term outcomes through precision oncology approaches [3, 14].

1.2 Molecular diversity of cancer biomarkers

Biomarkers are derived from diverse molecular entities, each offering unique cancer characterization, diagnosis, and management advantages. Their specificity and sensitivity vary depending on their molecular nature, making them indispensable in precision oncology.

- Proteins: Protein-based biomarkers are among the most well-established and widely used in clinical oncology. Examples include PSA (prostate cancer), CEA (colorectal cancer), and CA-125 (ovarian cancer), all of which can be detected in blood, urine, or tissues [6, 12, 15].

- Nucleic acids (DNA/RNA): Genetic and epigenetic alterations are robust cancer biomarkers. ctDNA is gaining attention as a non-invasive biomarker and disease monitoring and carries various modifications, including methylations, mutations, gene rearrangements, and microsatellite instability [16].

- Metabolites: Tumor cells undergo metabolic reprogramming, leading to distinct metabolic signatures that can be exploited as biomarkers. For instance, lactate dehydrogenase (LDH), a key enzyme in aerobic glycolysis, is frequently elevated in aggressive malignancies, including triple-negative breast cancer (TNBC) [17].

- Lipids: Emerging research in lipidomics has identified phospholipids and sphingolipids as potential biomarkers for tumor growth and metastasis, underscoring the role of altered lipid metabolism in cancer progression [18].

1.3 Biological fluids as biomarker sources

Biomarkers can be detected in various biological fluids, offering non-invasive or minimally invasive alternatives to traditional tissue biopsies [19]:

- Blood (Serum/Plasma): This is the most commonly used biofluid for biomarker detection. It contains circulating tumor cells (CTCs), cell-free DNA (cfDNA), exosomes [20], and protein markers such as AFP, CEA, and CA-19-9.

- Urine: Particularly useful for genitourinary cancers, with biomarkers such as Prostate Antigen 3 (PCA3) non-coding RNA for prostate cancer [21] and Nuclear matrix protein 22 (NMP22) for bladder cancer.

- Saliva: A promising biofluid for liquid biopsy, containing DNA, RNA, and proteins, including *KRAS* mRNA, which have been associated with pancreatic cancer detection [22].

- Cerebrospinal fluid (CSF): A valuable resource for detecting brain tumor biomarkers, including Glial fibrillary acidic protein (GFAP) in glioblastomas [23].

1.4 Technological advances driving biomarker discovery

Cutting-edge molecular technologies have significantly enhanced the development of cancer biomarkers, expanding the scope of their applications in clinical oncology.

- Next-generation sequencing (NGS) enables comprehensive genomic profiling, facilitating the identification of tumor-specific mutations, epigenetic alterations, and gene expression changes [5].

- Proteomics and mass spectrometry: Allow for large-scale protein-biomarker discovery and improve the detection of disease-specific proteins in biofluids [24].

- Liquid biopsy technologies: Enable minimally invasive detection and monitoring ctDNA, cfDNA, and extracellular vesicles (e.g. exossomes), transforming cancer diagnostics and monitoring [20].

- Single-cell sequencing provides unprecedented insights into tumor heterogeneity, allowing the analysis of the molecular landscape of individual cancer cells [25].

1.5 Challenges in translating biomarkers to clinical practice

Integrating biomarkers into routine clinical practice remains a multifaceted challenge despite significant advancements. Several key barriers must be overcome to ensure their successful clinical translation:

- Analytical validation and reproducibility: Biomarkers must demonstrate consistent performance across different patient populations, laboratories, and analytical platforms. Standardization of sample processing and data interpretation is crucial to ensure reproducibility [26].

- Clinical validation: Large-scale, well-controlled clinical trials are essential to establish a biomarker's predictive or prognostic utility and to determine its complementarity with existing diagnostic tools [27].

- Regulatory approval: Agencies such as the Food and Drug Administration (FDA) or EMA (European Medicines Agency) require extensive validation studies before approving biomarkers for clinical use, often resulting in delays in implementation [28].

- Cost-effectiveness and accessibility: Biomarkers must provide a significant clinical benefit relative to cost. While advanced techniques such as ctDNA sequencing show promise, high costs remain a barrier to widespread adoption [5].

- Tumor heterogeneity and disease evolution: Intratumoral molecular diversity complicates biomarker interpretation, and cancer progression can alter biomarker relevance over time [29].

2. The five most common cancer types worldwide

The five most common types of cancer worldwide, according to the latest GLOBOCAN 2022 estimates, are lung, breast, colorectal, prostate, and stomach cancers. These malignancies constitute a significant portion of the global cancer burden in terms of incidence and mortality, affecting millions of people annually [1].

Due to ongoing population growth and increasing urbanization, cancer global incidence will reach 35 million cases by the year 2050. This alarming project emphasizes the urgent need to invest in prevention, early detection, and equitable treatment strategies to mitigate its impact on public health worldwide [2].

2.1 Lung cancer

2.1.1 Epidemiology and risk factors

Lung cancer (LC) is the most common neoplasm, accounting for approximately 2.5 million cases in 2022, in addition to being the leading cause of cancer-related deaths, accounting for approximately 1.8 million deaths worldwide [1]. Smoking is the leading risk factor associated with the development of the disease, accounting for approximately 80% of cases. However, approximately 15% of smokers will develop LC throughout their lives, suggesting the existence of a genetic susceptibility that acts synergistically. Other risk factors include air pollution, exposure to asbestos, and family history [30].

Thanks to scientific advances in prevention, early detection, and treatments, mortality rates from CL have decreased in the last 5 years, while survival rates have increased considerably. Among these innovations, immunotherapies stand out, especially those based on immune checkpoint inhibitors. In the field of prevention, anti-smoking campaigns have represented an important strategy, as they have been quite effective in countries such as Australia and Brazil, which implemented public policies and educational programs that contributed to reducing the smoking population in these nations [31].

Generally asymptomatic in its early stages, LC is often diagnosed late, which contributes to its high mortality rate. When diagnosed early, LC can have a five-year survival rate of 40%. Approximately 70% of LC cases are diagnosed at more advanced stages, with a five-year survival rate of less than 12%. Low-dose spiral computed tomography (LDCT) is considered the standard method for early diagnosis of LC. Still, it has some disadvantages, such as a high false-positive rate and radiation exposure. To aid in diagnosis, clinicians investigate some molecular biomarkers in a solid biopsy to classify the molecular and histological subtype, define the therapeutic strategy, and predict prognosis [32].

2.1.2 Subtypes classification and biomarkers

Typically, LC can be subdivided into two main types: NSCLC, the most common and heterogeneous subtype, accounting for 85% of cases, and small cell carcinoma (SCLC), which accounts for 15% of cases, characterized by high aggressiveness and capacity for dissemination (metastasis). NSCLC can further be subdivided into three types: lung adenocarcinoma (LUAD), which originates from mucus-producing cells of the alveoli, the most common type among non-smokers; squamous cell carcinoma (SqCLC), which is strongly associated with smoking; and large cell carcinoma (LCLC), characterized by undifferentiated cells that can arise in any part of the lung [33].

The different subtypes of LC can be classified by immunohistochemistry by investigating a collection of protein biomarkers. Among the different types of NSCLC, positivity for the proteins Cytokeratin 7 (CK7) and Transcriptional termination factor 1 (TTF-1) in surgical specimens combined with negativity for p63, Cytokeratin ⅚ (CK5/6), and p40 characterizes the LUAD subtype. In contrast, these proteins' inverse pattern of expression characterizes the SqCCL subtype [33]. Another protein biomarker capable of differentiating these two subtypes is mucin, which is positive in LUAD and negative in SqCCL. As observed, LC is a highly heterogeneous disease, which makes the use of biomarkers essential for the classification of its subtypes in clinical practice. In addition, these biomarkers are essential for identifying patients who may benefit from targeted therapies and for helping predict prognosis. Some molecular biomarkers can be investigated in solid biopsy to aid in accurate diagnosis and define the treatments used in the therapeutic strategy [34].

The first molecular alterations identified and associated with LC were mutations in the gene encoding the EGFR protein and translocations in the Anaplastic lymphoma kinase (*ALK*) and cROS oncogene 1(*ROS1*)genes identified in solid biopsies and described as drivers for lung cancer. In addition to serving as diagnostic biomarkers, these alterations are targets of targeted therapies. In the case of EGFR mutations, the patient benefits from treatments with TKIs, such as erlotinib, gefitinib, and afatinib. Translocations in the *ALK* and *ROS1* genes can be targets of specific inhibitors such as ceritinib, alectinib, and crizotinib [4, 32]. New genetic and epigenetic alterations and gene expression patterns have been identified with the advancement of next-generation sequencing and other omics analysis techniques. They can currently be used as molecular biomarkers in clinical practice [35].

Obtaining tissue biopsies is often complicated and is an invasive procedure for the patient. Liquid biopsies have been used as a minimally invasive alternative for the diagnosis and monitoring of cancer patients, mainly through the use of blood samples to identify genetic mutations and epigenetic alterations related to cancer. Epigenetic alterations play a fundamental role in cancer biology, and many studies have demonstrated that these modifications can be identified in the cfDNA of cancer patients, more specifically ctDNA, which is released into the bloodstream by apoptotic tumor cells. Some alterations in DNA methylation have already been identified in the plasma of patients with LC and can be used as potential biomarkers for early diagnosis and prognosis. The methylation levels of the promoter region of the genes galactosilgalactosilxilosilproteína 3-beta-glucuronosyltransferase 2 (*B3GAT2*), Homeobox only protein X (*HOPX*), Homeobox D11 (*HOXD11*), *MIR1203*, myosin light chain 9 (*MYL9*), and Hepatic leukemia factor (*HLF*) are altered in patients with LC. These genes are related to tumor cell evasion of the immune system, tumor progression, and metastasis [36].

Identifying methylation of other genes in liquid biopsies can already be applied in clinical practice, such as altering methylation in the Short stature homeobox (*SHOX2*) gene to diagnose LC from plasma samples. Several clinical trials have already demonstrated that *SHOX2* increases the number of LC diagnoses when combined with histological and/or cytological tests and can be used as a strategy for early diagnosis [37]. Methylation of Ras-associated domain family 1A (*RASSF1A*) as a supplementary method for the diagnosis of LC from plasma and bronchial aspirate [38]. Methylation of the promoter region of the SRY-BOX transcription factor 17 (*SOX17*) gene has been used to predict clinical prognosis from plasma and sputum samples. *SOX17* acts as a negative regulator of the β-catenin pathway. Thus, patients who present higher methylation in the promoter region of this gene tend to exhibit increased activation of this signaling pathway, which may result in greater aggressiveness of the disease [39].

2.2 Breast cancer

2.2.1 Epidemiology and risk factors

Breast cancer (BC) is the most common neoplasm among women worldwide. In 2022, researchers estimated 2.3 million new cases, identifying it as the leading cause of cancer-related mortality in this group [1]. The main risk factors associated with BC include nulliparity, family history of the disease, genetic alterations, early menarche, late menopause, and obesity. Lifestyle changes, such as the adoption of Westernized dietary patterns, reduced physical activity, and increased obesity rates, constitute additional risk factors, particularly among postmenopausal women [40].

Screening asymptomatic individuals is essential for detecting tumors early, directly impacting patient survival. The primary BC screening strategies include mammography, recommended from the age of 40 [41]. Magnetic resonance imaging is indicated for women at high risk, such as those carrying BReast CAncer type 1 and type 2 (*BRCA1/BRCA2*) mutations or with a significant family history and should be performed annually in conjunction with mammography [42].

BC treatment is multimodal and depends on the stage of the disease, molecular subtype, and individual patient characteristics. In general, it includes surgery (e.g., mastectomy), radiotherapy or brachytherapy, chemotherapy (administered in different settings, such as adjuvant, neoadjuvant, or palliative), hormonal therapy, targeted therapies, and immunotherapy. Immunotherapy, for instance, is indicated for triple-negative breast cancer (TNBC) cases that exhibit PD-L1 expression or MSI-H) [43]. Despite well-established screening, diagnostic, and treatment strategies, researchers continue to develop biomarkers to improve early detection, risk stratification, and therapeutic personalization. Integrating precision medicine will likely enhance clinical outcomes.

2.2.2 Subtypes classification and biomarkers

Clinicians have incorporated several biomarkers into clinical practice for BC diagnosis and monitoring. Among the key predictive biomarkers are hormone receptors, such as the estrogen receptor (ER), progesterone receptor (PR), and human HER2, which are fundamental for the molecular classification of BC. These markers classify tumors into four major subtypes: Luminal A, Luminal B, HER2-positive (HER2+), and TNBC [44, 45].

TNBC is considered the subtype with the poorest prognosis due to its heterogeneity and lack of specific targeted therapies. However, gene expression profiling studies have identified six distinct molecular subtypes within TNBC: Basal-like 1, Basal-like 2, Mesenchymal, Mesenchymal Stem-like (MSL), Immunomodulatory, and Luminal Androgen Receptor [46]. This classification holds the potential to guide more targeted therapeutic approaches. Studies have shown that women with higher proportions of African genetic ancestry are more likely to be diagnosed with aggressive BC subtypes, such as TNBC, and often at more advanced stages. A combination of genetic, socioeconomic, and systemic factors influences this disparity. A higher percentage of West African ancestry correlates with shorter disease-free survival in hormone receptor-positive BC cases [47, 48].

HER2 gene amplification drives a more aggressive tumor phenotype in HER2-positive BC. Historically, this subtype was associated with a poor prognosis; however, the development of targeted therapies has revolutionized its management, significantly improving patient survival. Among the primary agents used are trastuzumab (Herceptin®), pertuzumab (Perjeta®), and ado-trastuzumab emtansine (Kadcyla®), the latter being indicated for treatment-resistant disease [49].

Monitoring biomarkers, such as CEA, Cancer Antigen 15-3 (CA15-3), and Cancer Antigen 27-29 (CA27-29), are widely utilized to assess recurrence and metastasis. These biomarkers are glycoproteins, and their serum levels increase in advanced disease, allowing for the monitoring of therapeutic response [50–52].

Mutations in the BRCA1 and BRCA2 genes serve as predisposition biomarkers strongly associated with an elevated risk of breast and ovarian cancer. Women harboring pathogenic mutations in these genes have a significantly increased lifetime risk of developing these malignancies, justifying the implementation of personalized preventive measures [53].

Patients also benefit from multigene panels, such as Oncotype DX (developed by Genomic Health) and MammaPrint (developed by Agendia), which evaluate the transcriptional expression of multiple biomarkers, assisting in prognostic stratification and therapeutic decision-making. NanoString Technologies developed the Prosigna test (PAM50) to analyze the expression of 50 genes at the mRNA level, generating a risk score from 0 to 100. This score helps assess ER-positive patients undergoing endocrine therapy or adjuvant chemotherapy. The FDA approves these panels, which are widely used in clinical practice to guide personalized treatment decisions in breast cancer care [54].

Among the best-validated prognostic biomarkers forBC care Urokinase plasminogen activator (uPA) and its inhibitor, Plasminogen activator inhibitor-1 (PAI-1), particularly in patients with node-negative disease. These proteolytic enzymes play a crucial role in tumor invasion and metastasis, and high levels are associated with poor prognosis. PAI-1 binds to uPA, promoting receptor internalization and inactivation, leading to cell detachment from the extracellular matrix. Additionally, PAI-1 inhibits uPA activity and interacts with biological ligands, contributing to tissue remodeling and cell migration [55].

UPA/PAI-1 is clinically used as a prognostic biomarker to guide risk stratification and therapeutic decisions. Patients with high levels of uPA/PAI-1 face an increased risk of recurrence, which may indicate the need for adjuvant chemotherapy in early-stage BC. Conversely, low levels of uPA/PAI-1 are associated with a more favorable prognosis, allowing some patients to avoid unnecessary chemotherapy. However, its clinical implementation remains limited, primarily due to the requirement for fresh tumor samples and restricted availability in routine pathology laboratories. Additionally, the emergence of genomic signatures such as Oncotype DX and MammaPrint has provided more comprehensive molecular profiling, reducing the widespread use of uPA/PAI-1 in clinical practice [55–57].

Microbiome assessment, including breast tissue microbiome, has emerged as a promising approach to identifying novel biomarkers. Researchers have recently identified the microbiome as a hallmark of cancer due to its role in modulating tumor progression through chronic inflammation, immune response regulation, and alterations in cellular metabolism. The microbiome represents a potential new therapeutic target in precision oncology. Advances in sequencing technologies have significantly enhanced the discovery of novel biomarkers, enabling more precise risk stratification and personalized treatment strategies [58, 59].

2.3 Colorectal cancer

2.3.1 Epidemiology and risk factors

Colorectal cancer (CRC) is one of the main diseases affecting the digestive tract, being the third most common type of cancer worldwide and the second leading cause of cancer-related deaths [1] The main risk factors for CRC include advanced age, family history, genetic syndromes such as Familial Adenomatous Polyposis and Lynch Syndrome, poor diet, and alcohol/tobacco use. The primary reason for the high mortality rate is the difficulty of early diagnosis, as there are no clinical signs of the disease in its initial stages, and the tumor's incubation period is extremely slow. As a result, tumor detection usually occurs when it is already at an advanced stage, leading to a worse prognosis [60]. For this reason, using biomarkers that can assist in earlier diagnosis is extremely necessary.

Currently, colonoscopy is considered the gold standard for diagnosing and screening CRC [60]. However, several countries have already approved using the Septin-9 (*SEPT9*) gene methylation test as a non-invasive alternative for the early diagnosis of CRC, especially in patients with contraindications for colonoscopy. This epigenetic marker has high sensitivity, particularly in the early stages of the disease, and can be detected through plasma samples rich in cfDNA [61]. Another well-known biomarker for CRC is CEA, detected in blood serum and commonly used to monitor disease progression. The sensitivity of CEA is quite limited in the early stages of the tumor, making it a poor marker for early diagnosis [13]. However, as the tumor progresses, CEA levels increase, enhancing both sensitivity and specificity. Therefore, since patients with this tumor exhibit high CEA levels, a decrease in these levels during therapy may indicate a positive response to treatment. Persistent or recurrent increases in CEA levels may suggest disease progression, making it also the primary biomarker for recurrence [62].

2.3.2 Subtypes classification and biomarkers

However, colorectal tumors are highly heterogeneous, with different classifications and distinct molecular characteristics, prognoses, and treatments, necessitating biomarkers with greater specificity. CRC can be divided, based on molecular classification, into four main subtypes: CMS1 (immunogenic), CMS2 (canonical), CMS3 (metabolic), and CMS4 (mesenchymal) [63].

CMS1 tumors generally have a better prognosis and are characterized by MSI-H. They may also exhibit Humam mutL homolog 1 (hMLH1) hypermethylation, with these molecules being the primary biomarkers for identifying this subtype. hMLH1 hypermethylation is associated with sporadic mutations, while MSI-H without this hypermethylation is more commonly linked to hereditary mutations from Lynch syndrome. Another widely used biomarker is BRAF, which is frequently mutated in CMS1, confirming the identification of this subtype and helping to differentiate it from others. As for prognostic and therapeutic targeting biomarkers, PD-L1 protein expression is commonly used in clinical practice for this subtype, determining the use of immunotherapy in patients [63, 64].

CMS2 tumors are the most common and are characterized by chromosomal instability (CIN), with the main identification biomarkers are mutations in Adenomatous polyposis coli (*APC*) and *TP53* genes and the activation of Wnt and Myc signaling pathways. The *TP53* gene mutations frequently observed in this subtype can also serve as prognostic biomarkers, as they are associated with greater tumor aggressiveness [63, 65].

CMS3 tumors exhibit metabolic dysregulation and are generally associated with a poor prognosis. The main identification biomarkers for this subtype are mutations in the *KRAS* gene and the activation of the receptor tyrosine kinase (RTK) and mitogen-activated protein kinase (MAPK) pathways. *KRAS* is a gene encoding a GTPase involved in regulating cell growth and division; therefore, mutations can lead to uncontrolled tumor growth and resistance to apoptosis. Additionally, patients with *KRAS* mutations are resistant to therapies involving EGFR inhibitors, such as cetuximab, making treatment with this medication unfeasible. Thus, *KRAS* can also be used in clinical practice as a biomarker for prognosis and therapeutic targeting [63, 66].

CMS4 tumors are characterized by increased expression of genes involved in epithelial-mesenchymal transition (EMT), having a greater propensity for metastasis or recurrence, making this the subtype with the worst prognosis. Among the biomarkers used for identification are key genes associated with mesenchymal activation, such as Vimnentin (*VIM*), Zinc finger E-Box binding homeobox 1 (*ZEB1*), and Snail family transcriptional repressor (*SNAI1*). These genes can also be used as prognostic biomarkers, along with Transforming growth factor beta (TGF-β) and Interleukin 6 (IL-6), whose high expression leads to greater EMT activation and disease progression [13, 63].

2.4 Prostate cancer

2.4.1 Epidemiology, risk factors and screening

Prostate cancer is one of the most prevalent cancers among men, with an estimated 1.4 million new cases in 2022, accounting for 7.3% of cancer-related deaths in men [1]. Screening strategies for prostate cancer are more limited compared to breast cancer. Prostate epithelial cells produce PSA, a serine protease detectable in the blood. Clinicians widely use elevated PSA levels as a screening biomarker for prostate cancer diagnosis and monitoring. However, elevated PSA can be associated with benign conditions such as benign prostatic hyperplasia and prostatitis, leading to false positives [67].

Additionally, some malignant prostate tumors exhibit low PSA levels, resulting in false negatives. Therefore, other tests such as a digital rectal examination, prostate ultrasound, and biopsy may be associated with prostate cancer screening and diagnosis. Given this scenario, there is a clear need for more effective biomarkers for screening and diagnosing this type of cancer [68].

Understanding the risk factors associated with the disease is of great importance. Non-modifiable risk factors for prostate cancer include age, race, family history, and germline mutations. In contrast, modifiable risk factors such as metabolic syndrome, obesity, and smoking, as well as environmental factors, are also linked to the disease's etiology [69, 70].

Regarding the clinical approach to prostate cancer, it is still predominantly based on clinical and histopathological criteria, evaluating PSA levels, Gleason score (histological grade), and clinical staging (TNM). However, molecular biomarkers have played an increasing role, especially in advanced or treatment-resistant cases, although there is still no consensus on molecular subtypes in the literature [71]. In terms of therapy, several main treatments are well-established, including radical prostatectomy, cryotherapy (which may present complications such as urinary incontinence and erectile dysfunction), radiation therapy, brachytherapy, and chemotherapy [72].

Most cases of prostate cancer are androgen-dependent. This subtype is characterized by its reliance on androgen signaling for growth and survival. Alterations in DNA repair genes such as Ataxia telangiectasia mutated (*ATM*), *BRCA1*, *BRCA2*, and Checkpoint kinase 2 (*CHEK2*) are associated with a higher risk of prostate cancer development, as well as more aggressive tumors that respond to therapies involving poly(ADP-ribose) polymerase (PARP) inhibitors. Men of African ancestry have genetic variants that predispose them to more aggressive prostate cancer. Therefore, the proportions of genetic ancestry, epigenetic, and environmental factors such as migration and dietary patterns are considered contributing factors [67, 73].

2.4.2 Subtypes classification and biomarkers

Prostate cancer exhibits various epigenetic alterations, including aberrant hypermethylation in CpG promoter islands, DNA hypomethylation, histone acetylation that may lead to super-enhancer formation, and deregulated histone methylation. Among these alterations, aberrant hypermethylation of promoter regions can impact repair, cell cycle regulation, and apoptosis genes. Hypermethylation of the (glutathione S-transferase Pi 1(*GSTP1*)) gene is one of the most common epigenetic events in prostate cancer, promoting gene silencing and predominantly occurring in the promoter region in CpG islands. Present in approximately 90% of prostate adenocarcinoma cases, GSTP1 silencing through methylation is considered an early event in the development of this type of cancer. Thus, GSTP1 hypermethylation in prostate samples can serve as a diagnostic biomarker, as it is detected explicitly in prostate cancer and prostatic intraepithelial neoplasia but not in normal or benign tissues [74].

Transmembrane serine protease 2 – ETS-related gene (TMPRSS2-ERG), a gene fusion resulting in overexpression of the ERG oncogene, is present in approximately 50% of prostate cancer cases. This gene fusion is associated with more aggressive tumors, typically in cases that are castration-resistant and lack approved specific therapies. However, it has low sensitivity [75].

Clinicians use biomarkers such as the 4Kscore, Prostate Health Index (PHI), and PCA3 to diagnose prostate cancer and guide treatment decisions. Their applications are specific and used in different clinical contexts, especially where traditional PSA may not be sufficient. The 4Kscore combines four blood biomarkers: total PSA (tPSA), free PSA (fPSA), intact PSA, and human kallikrein 2 (hK2), along with clinical factors such as age, biopsy history, and digital rectal exam findings. Clinicians use this test to assess the risk of aggressive prostate cancer (high-grade, Gleason ≥7) in men with elevated PSA or suspicious rectal exam results. It aids in risk stratification and guides decisions on needing a biopsy [76, 77].

The PHI is a calculation that combines the values of total PSA (tPSA), free PSA (fPSA), and proPSA (a specific form of PSA associated with prostate cancer). In diagnosis, it improves the accuracy of traditional PSA to predict the likelihood of prostate cancer, especially in men with PSA levels between 2 and 10 ng/mL. Like the 4Kscore, it is evaluated from blood samples and may help avoid unnecessary biopsies and assist in assessing the risk of cancer progression in patients under active surveillance. Clinicians use it as a complementary tool to traditional PSA [78]. PCA3, a non-coding messenger RNA, is overexpressed in more than 95% of prostate tumors. It is detected in urine following a prostate massage. Diagnosis helps improve the specificity of traditional PSA, especially in men with elevated PSA and previous negative biopsies. PCA3 is used in clinical practice as a complementary test to PSA, particularly in cases of last negative biopsies [79].

Macrophage scavenger receptor 1 (*MSR1*) may be considered a genetic susceptibility biomarker for prostate cancer, particularly in contexts of hereditary prostate cancer. However, due to its variable penetrance, genetic heterogeneity, and lack of consensus in different populations, it is not widely used in current clinical practice [80].

The transcription factorHomeobox B 13 (*HOXB13*)reduces prostate cancer growth and androgen receptor-mediated activity. The common variant (rs339331) enhances *HOXB13* binding to an enhancer, strengthening its regulatory role [67]. However, *HOXB13* variants correlate with an increased risk of aggressive and early-onset prostate cancer [81].

Genomic panels are playing an increasing role in personalizing prostate cancer treatment, contributing to better diagnosis, prognosis, and therapeutic decision-making. Oncotype DX GPS (Genomic Prostate Score), developed by Genomic Health, is one of the most widely used tests. It evaluates the expression of 17 genes to estimate the risk of disease progression in patients with low- and intermediate-risk prostate cancer. This FDA-approved test aids in deciding between active surveillance and definitive treatment and is widely used in clinical practice [82].

Prolaris, developed by Myriad Genetics, measures the expression of cell cycle-related genes to predict tumor aggressiveness and the risk of metastatic progression. It helps in risk stratification and decision-making about active treatment, and it is also widely used in clinical practice. Decipher, developed by GenomeDx Biosciences, is based on transcriptome analysis to provide a prognostic score for patients undergoing radical prostatectomy, estimating the risk of biochemical recurrence and metastasis. This panel also guides adjuvant therapy and is available for clinical use with regulatory approval [82].

ConfirmMDx, developed by MDxHealth, is an epigenetic test that assesses gene hypermethylation in negative prostate biopsies, helping to reduce false negatives and identify patients who may need repeat biopsies. Finally, ExoDx Prostate (EPI), from Exosome Diagnostics, is a non-invasive test based on extracellular RNA found in urine, used to differentiate low- and high-risk cancers, helping to avoid unnecessary biopsies. All these tests have regulatory approval and are widely used in clinical practice to guide prostate cancer treatment [83].

2.5 Stomach cancer

2.5.1 Epidemiology and risk factors

Gastric cancer (GC), also known as stomach cancer, is the fifth most common type of tumor in terms of incidence and mortality worldwide [1]. Among the main risk factors for the disease are infection with the bacterium *Helicobacter pylori* (*H. pylori*), as well as poor diet, tobacco use, and genetic/hereditary factors. The low overall survival rate of patients with GC is due to the advanced stage at which the tumor is usually detected, often already in the process of metastasis [84]. Therefore, screening and early diagnosis are crucial to improving patient prognosis.

Currently, endoscopy is considered the gold standard for GC screening, as it allows for direct visualization of the stomach's inner lining and the collection of biopsies for histopathological analysis. However, it has some limitations, such as insufficient sensitivity and specificity for detecting lesions at early stages [85]. Additionally, it is considered an invasive procedure that requires specialized and high-tech infrastructure. As a result, the search for non-invasive biomarkers has gained prominence, but no diagnostic biomarkers have yet been identified for clinical use.

2.5.2 Subtypes classification and biomarkers

Some potential GC biomarkers currently under investigation include miRNAs, ctDNA, extracellular vesicles (exosomes), and proteins. All of these molecules can be detected through liquid biopsy, which is considered less invasive [85]. Additionally, epigenetic studies have explored DNA methylation of genes as a potential biomarker for the early detection of GC, especially in cases associated with *H. pylori* infection. DNA methylation is one of the main epigenetic changes this pathogen induces when it infects the gastric mucosa, potentially activating crucial signaling pathways for tumor development, such as the Fibroblast growth factor receptor 4 (*FGFR4*) and Signal transducer and activator of transcription 3 (STAT3) pathways [85].

GC is also considered a highly heterogeneous type of cancer. It is histologically classified by Lauren into three main types: (1) Intestinal – characterized by glandular cells, which tend to grow in a more localized manner and have a better prognosis; (2) Diffuse – marked by signet ring cells, which have a worse prognosis and a higher risk of metastasis; and (3) Mixed – which presents both intestinal-type and diffuse-type cells, with the prognosis depending on the proportion of each type [86]. Additionally, GC is classified by The Cancer Genome Atlas (TCGA) into four main molecular subtypes: Epstein-Barr virus-associated (EBV-positive), MSI-H, genomically stable (GS), and chromosomal instability (CIN) [87].

EBV-positive tumors exhibit extreme DNA hypermethylation, particularly in the promoter region of the Cyclin-dependent kinase inhibitor 2A (*CDKN2A*) gene, as well as frequent mutations in Phosphatidylinositol-4,5-bisphosphate 3-kinase catalytic subunit alpha gene (*PIK3CA*), which has directed therapeutic research toward epigenetic modulation and the PI3 kinase pathway. Additionally, they overexpress PD-L1/2, leading to reduced responsiveness to immunotherapy [87, 88]. MSI-H tumors also show high hypermethylation, typically observed in the promoter region of the MutL homolog 1 (*MLH1*) gene, which compromises the DNA repair system, resulting in an increased mutation rate. These tumors are considered to have a better prognosis and are highly responsive to immunotherapy, with MSI-H already being used as a clinical biomarker [87, 89]. On the other hand, GS tumors, commonly observed in the diffuse histological type, are characterized by mutations in the Cadherin 1 (*CDH1*) and Ras homolog family member A (*RHOA*) genes, which lead to loss of cell adhesion and increased metastatic potential, respectively, making this subtype one of the worst prognoses [87, 90]. Finally, CIN tumors, typically of the intestinal histological type, exhibit a high frequency of chromosome number and structure changes. They are characterized by silencing tumor suppressor genes, such as TP53, and the amplification of HER-2, EGFR, and/or Fibroblast growth factor receptor 2 (*FGFR2*) genes, which are also quite common. These features can influence therapeutic targeting and the prognosis of the disease [87, 91].

Among these discoveries, only the MSI-H/dMMR test is currently used in clinical practice as a biomarker, along with HER-2, which is used as a prognostic biomarker [92]. All other potential biomarkers are still under research and/or optimization.

Despite significant advances in biomarker research and development for clinical applications, several challenges remain in oncology precision medicine. Problems such as reproducibility, specificity, technical complexity, and intra- and intertumoral variability hinder the validation of effective biomarkers. Nevertheless, biomarkers have been validated and integrated into clinical practice, significantly advancing cancer diagnosis, prognosis, and treatment, highlighting the ongoing importance of research and innovation (**Figure 2**; **Table 1**).

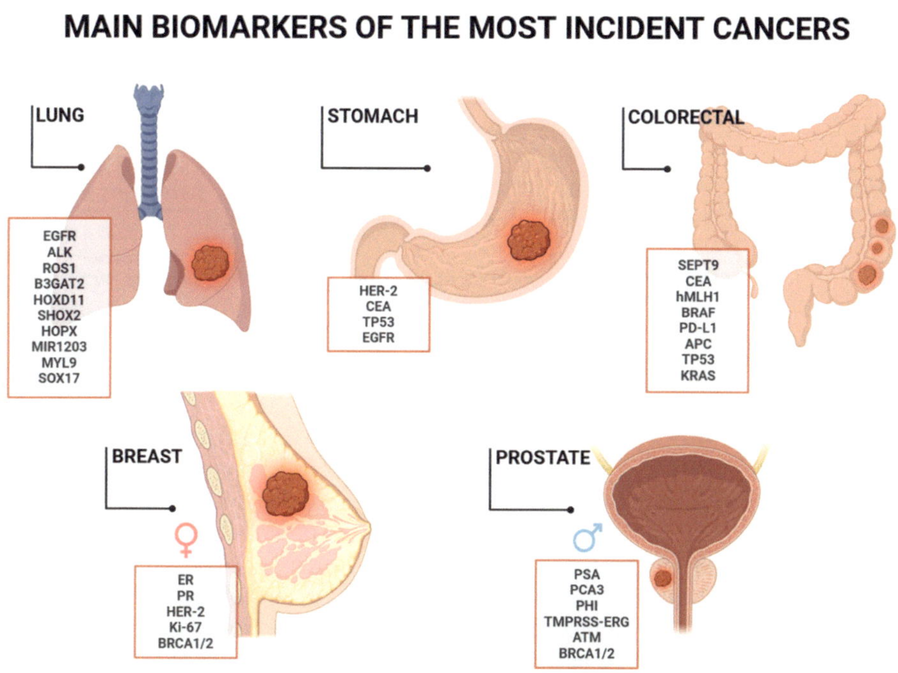

Figure 2.
Molecular biomarkers associated with the most prevalent cancers. The figure illustrates lung, stomach, colorectal, breast, and prostate cancers, highlighting key molecular biomarkers for each organ.

Biomarker	Type of cancer	Sample	Molecular alteration	Function
ALK, ROS1	Lung	Tissue	Translocation	Diagnosis
EGFR	Lung	Tissue/ Blood	Mutation	Diagnosis, Treatment
	Gastric	Tissue	Overexpression	Prognosis and Treatment
B3GAT2, HOXD11, SHOX2, HOPX, MIR1203, MYL9	Lung	Blood	Methylation	Diagnosis
SOX17	Lung	Blood	Methylation	Diagnosis and Prognosis
MUCIN	Lung	Tissue	Overexpression	Diagnosis
ER	Breast	Tissue	Overexpression	Treatment and Subtype Identification
PR	Breast	Tissue	Overexpression	Treatment and Subtype Identification
HER-2	Breast	Tissue	Overexpression/ Amplification	Treatment and Subtype Identification
	Gastric	Tissue	Overexpression	Treatment and Subtype Identification
Ki-67	Breast	Tissue	Overexpression	Prognosis, Treatment and Subtype Identification
BRCA1/2	Breast	Blood	Mutation	Predisposition
PSA	Prostate	Blood	Amplification	Diagnosis and Monitoring
SEPT9	Colorectal	Blood	Methylation	Diagnosis
CEA	Colorectal Gastric	Blood	Amplification	Monitoring
hMLH1	Colorectal	Blood	Methylation	Subtype Identification
BRAF	Colorectal	Blood	Mutation	Prognosis and Subtype Identification

Table 1.
Biomarkers in cancer.

3. Integration of biomarkers into precision medicine strategies

The future of oncology is intricately linked to the continuous evolution of biomarker-driven precision medicine. Advances in multiomic profiling-integrating genomic, transcriptomic, proteomic, and metabolomic data are refining biomarker discovery and improving diagnostic and prognostic accuracy. As cancer research progresses, the ability to personalize treatment based on biomarker signatures will increasingly lead to improved patient outcomes and minimize treatment-related toxicity [5].

Integrating artificial intelligence (AI) and machine learning (ML) will revolutionize biomarker identification and application. AI-driven algorithms can analyze vast datasets and identify complex biomarker patterns to predict patient therapy responses. These advancements will enable oncologists to make data-driven treatment decisions, significantly improving the effectiveness of precision medicine [93].

3.1 Future perspectives and directions in cancer research

The development of next-generation liquid biopsy technologies is the future direction of biomarker research [5]. New techniques advanced in single-cell sequencing, extracellular vesicle analysis, and enhanced detection ctDNA are leading the way for earlier cancer detection, monitoring, and treatment adaptation. These innovations will further decrease the dependence on invasive tissue biopsies, making precision medicine in oncology more accessible and efficient.

Another transformative trend is the integration of immune-related biomarkers in immunotherapy strategies. The identification of novel immune checkpoints, tumor microenvironment signatures, and microbiome interactions will expand the range of patients who can benefit from immunotherapies. The personalization of immune-based treatments using predictive biomarkers will be crucial in addressing therapy resistance and improving response rates in traditionally unresponsive tumor types [94].

Furthermore, the discovery of epigenetic biomarkers is expected to increase, particularly in understanding tumor plasticity and treatment resistance. DNA methylation signature, non-coding RNA profile, and histone modifications will offer insights into tumor evolution, allowing for more effective targeting of aggressive and adaptive cancer subtypes [95].

Despite these promising innovations, challenges remain in regimenting biomarker implementation in clinical practice. Regulatory approval processes, cost barriers, and the need for robust validation in large-scale clinical trials must be addressed to ensure the widespread adoption of biomarker-driven therapies. Collaborative efforts among research institutions, pharmaceutical companies, and regulatory agencies will be essential in overcoming these obstacles [96].

4. Conclusion

In conclusion, the future of oncology will be shaped by integrating cutting-edge biomarker technologies into precision medicine frameworks. Advances in liquid biopsies, AI-driven analytics, immune profiling, and epigenetics will continue to refine cancer detection, prognosis, and treatment selection. As research progresses, a multi-disciplinary approach combining computational biology, molecular oncology, and clinical expertise will be critical in translating these innovations into tangible improvements in patient care, ultimately reducing cancer mortality and enhancing long-term survival.

Conflict of interest

The authors declare no conflict of interest.

Author details

Tatiana de Almeida Simão[1*], Jennifer Vieira Gomes[1], Diego José Gomes de Paula[2] and Suzana Pinheiro de Oliveira Ribeiro[1]

1 State University of Rio de Janeiro, Rio de Janeiro, Brazil

2 National Cancer Institute, Rio de Janeiro, Brazil

*Address all correspondence to: tasimão@gmail.com

References

[1] Bray F, Laversanne M, Sung H, Ferlay J, Siegel RL, Soerjomataram I, et al. Global cancer statistics 2022: GLOBOCAN estimates of incidence and mortality worldwide for 36 cancers in 185 countries. CA: A Cancer Journal for Clinicians. 2024;**74**(3):229-263. DOI: 10.3322/caac.21834

[2] Ferlay J, Ervik M, Lam F, Laversanne M, Colombet M, Mery L, et al. Global Cancer Observatory: Cancer Today (Version 1.1). Lyon, France: International Agency for Research on Cancer; 2024. Available from: https://gco.iarc.who.int/today

[3] Zhou Y, Tao L, Qiu J, Xu J, Yang X, Zhang Y, et al. Tumor biomarkers for diagnosis, prognosis and targeted therapy. Signal Transduction and Targeted Therapy. 2024;**9**(1):132. DOI: 10.1038/s41392-024-01823-2

[4] National Cancer Institute. Cancer Terms Dictionary. Available from: https://www.cancer.gov/publications/dictionaries/cancer-terms [Accessed: February 27, 2025]

[5] Passaro A, Al Bakir M, Hamilton EG, Diehn M, André F, Roy-Chowdhuri S, et al. Cancer biomarkers: Emerging trends and clinical implications for personalized treatment. Cell. 2024;**187**(7):1617-1635. DOI: 10.1016/j.cell.2024.02.041

[6] Lilja H, Ulmert D, Vickers AJ. Prostate-specific antigen and prostate cancer: Prediction, detection, and monitoring. Nature Reviews. Cancer. 2008;**8**(4):268-278. DOI: 10.1038/nrc2351

[7] Tsuchiya N, Sawada Y, Endo I, Saito K, Uemura Y, Nakatsura T. Biomarkers for the early diagnosis of hepatocellular carcinoma. World Journal of Gastroenterology. 2015;**21**(37):10573-10583. DOI: 10.3748/wjg.v21.i37.10573

[8] Slamon DJ, Clark GM, Wong SG, Levin WJ, Ullrich A, McGuire WL. Human breast cancer: Correlation of relapse and survival with amplification of the HER-2/neu oncogene. Science. 1987;**235**(4785):177-182. DOI: 10.1126/science.3798106

[9] Olivier M, Hollstein M, Hainaut P. TP53 mutations in human cancers: Origins, consequences, and clinical use. Cold Spring Harbor Perspectives in Biology. 2010;**2**(1):a001008. DOI: 10.1101/cshperspect.a001008

[10] Mok TS, Wu YL, Thongprasert S, Yang CH, Chu DT, Saijo N, et al. Gefitinib or carboplatin–paclitaxel in pulmonary adenocarcinoma. The New England Journal of Medicine. 2009;**361**(10):947-957. DOI: 10.1056/NEJMoa0810699

[11] Garon EB, Rizvi NA, Hui R, Leighl N, Balmanoukian AS, Eder JP, et al. Pembrolizumab for the treatment of non–small-cell lung cancer. The New England Journal of Medicine. 2015;**372**(21):2018-2028. DOI: 10.1056/NEJMoa1501824

[12] Nicholson BD, Shinkins B, Pathiraja I, Roberts NW, James TJ, Mallett S, et al. Blood CEA levels for detecting recurrent colorectal cancer. Cochrane Database of Systematic Reviews. 2015:CD011134, 1-27. DOI: 10.1002/14651858.CD011134.pub2

[13] Kamel F, Eltarhoni K, Nisar P, Soloviev M. Colorectal cancer diagnosis: The obstacles we face in determining a non-invasive test and current advances in biomarker detection. Cancers (Basel).

2022;**14**(8):1889. DOI: 10.3390/cancers14081889

[14] Diehl F, Schmidt K, Choti MA, Romans K, Goodman S, Li M, et al. Circulating mutant DNA to assess tumor dynamics. Nature Medicine. 2008;**14**(9):985-990. DOI: 10.1038/nm.1789

[15] Zhang M, Cheng S, Jin Y, Zhao Y, Wang Y. Roles of CA125 in diagnosis, prediction, and oncogenesis of ovarian cancer. Biochimica Et Biophysica Acta. Reviews on Cancer. 2021;**1875**(2):188503. DOI: 10.1016/j.bbcan.2021.188503

[16] Mishra M, Ahmed R, Das DK, Das Pramanik D, Dash SK, Pramanik A. Recent advancements in the application of circulating tumor DNA as biomarkers for early detection of cancers. ACS Biomaterials Science and Engineering. 2024;**10**(8):4740-4756. DOI: 10.1021/acsbiomaterials.4c00606

[17] Dong T, Liu Z, Xuan Q, Wang Z, Ma W, Zhang Q. Tumor LDH-A expression and serum LDH status are two metabolic predictors for triple negative breast cancer brain metastasis. Scientific Reports. 2017;**7**:6069. DOI: 10.1038/s41598-017-06378-7

[18] Pan M, Qin C, Han X. Lipid metabolism and lipidomics applications in cancer research. Advances in Experimental Medicine and Biology. 2021;**1316**:1-24. DOI: 10.1007/978-981-33-6785-2_1

[19] Domínguez-Vigil IG, Moreno-Martínez AK, Wang JY, Roehrl MHA, Barrera-Saldaña HA. The dawn of the liquid biopsy in the fight against cancer. Oncotarget. 2018;**9**:2912-2922. DOI: 10.18632/oncotarget.23131

[20] Batool SM, Yekula A, Khanna P, Hsia T, Gamblin AS, Castro CM, et al. The liquid biopsy consortium: Challenges and opportunities for early cancer detection and monitoring. Cell Reports Medicine. 2023;**4**(10):101198. DOI: 10.1016/j.xcrm.2023.101198

[21] Hessels D, Gunnewiek JMK, van Oort I, Karthaus HF, van Leenders GJ, van Balken B, et al. DD3(PCA3)-based molecular urine analysis for the diagnosis of prostate cancer. European Urology. 2003;**44**(1):8-16. DOI: 10.1016/j.urology.2006.12.014

[22] Zhang L, Farrell JJ, Zhou H, Elashoff D, Akin D, Park NH, et al. Salivary transcriptomic biomarkers for detection of resectable pancreatic cancer. Gastroenterology. 2010;**138**(3):949-57.e1-7. DOI: 10.1053/j.gastro.2009.11.010

[23] Xiao F, Lv S, Zong Z, Wu L, Tang X, Kuang W, et al. Cerebrospinal fluid biomarkers for brain tumor detection: Clinical roles and current progress. American Journal of Translational Research. 2020;**12**(4):1379-1396

[24] Sarhadi VK, Armengol G. Molecular biomarkers in cancer. Biomolecules. 2022;**12**(8):1021. DOI: 10.3390/biom12081021

[25] Navin N, Hicks J. Future medical applications of single-cell sequencing in cancer. Genome Medicine. 2011;**3**(5):31. DOI: 10.1186/gm247

[26] Moore HM, Kelly AB, Jewell SD, McShane LM, Clark DP, Greenspan R, et al. Biospecimen reporting for improved study quality (BRISQ). Journal of Proteome Research. 2011;**10**:3429-3438. DOI: 10.1021/pr200021n

[27] Ransohoff DF. How to improve reliability and efficiency of research about molecular markers: Roles of phases, guidelines, and study design. Journal of Clinical Epidemiology. 2007;**60**:1205-1219

[28] FDA-NIH Biomarker Working Group. BEST (Biomarkers, EndpointS, and Other Tools) Resource. Silver Spring (MD): Food and Drug Administration (US); 2016. Update in 2025

[29] McGranahan N, Swanton C. Clonal heterogeneity and tumor evolution: Past, present, and the future. Cell. 2017;**168**(4):613-628. DOI: 10.1016/j.cell.2017.01.018

[30] Siddiqui F, Vaqar S, Siddiqui AH. Lung cancer. [updated 2023 may 8]. In: StatPearls. Treasure Island (FL): StatPearls Publishing; 2024

[31] Schenk EL, Patil T, Pacheco J, Bunn PA Jr. 2020 innovation-based optimism for lung cancer outcomes. The Oncologist. 2021;**26**(3):e454-e472. DOI: 10.1002/onco.13590

[32] Saller JJ, Boyle TA. Molecular pathology of lung cancer. Cold Spring Harbor Perspectives in Medicine. 2022;**12**(3):a037812. DOI: 10.1101/cshperspect.a037812

[33] Adams SJ, Stone E, Baldwin DR, Vliegenthart R, Lee P, Fintelmann F. Lung cancer screening. Lancet. 2023;**401**(10374):390-408. DOI: 10.1016/S0140-6736(22)01694-4

[34] Siddique F, Shebata M, Ghazal M, Contractor S, El-Baz A. Lung cancer subtyping: A short review. Cancers (Basel). 2024;**16**(15):2643. DOI: 10.3390/cancers16152643

[35] Li W, Liu JB, Hou LK, Yu F, Zhang J, Wu W, et al. Liquid biopsy in lung cancer: Significance in diagnostics, prediction, and treatment monitoring. Molecular Cancer. 2022;**21**(1):25. DOI: 10.1186/s12943-022-01505-z

[36] Li P, Liu S, Du L, Mohseni G, Zhang Y, Wang C. Liquid biopsies based on DNA methylation as biomarkers for the detection and prognosis of lung cancer. Clinical Epigenetics. 2022;**14**(1):118. DOI: 10.1186/s13148-022-01337-0

[37] Song L, Yu H, Li Y. Diagnosis of lung cancer by SHOX2 gene methylation assay. Molecular Diagnosis and Therapy. 2015;**19**:159-167. DOI: 10.1007/s40291-015-0144-5

[38] Chen XP, He SX, Chen MY, Chen FB, Wu P, Shi P, et al. Meta-analysis of the accuracy for RASSF1A methylation in bronchial aspirates for the diagnosis of lung cancer. PLoS One. 2024;**19**(7):e0299447. DOI: 10.1371/journal.pone.0299447

[39] Balgkouranidou I, Chimonidou M, Milaki G, Tsaroucha E, Kakolyris S, Georgoulias V, et al. SOX17 promoter methylation in plasma circulating tumor DNA of patients with non-small cell lung cancer. Clinical Chemistry and Laboratory Medicine. 2016;**54**(8):1385-1393. DOI: 10.1515/cclm-2015-0776

[40] American Cancer Society. Breast Cancer Risk and Prevention: Risk Factors. 2023. Available from: https://www.cancer.org/cancer/breast-cancer/risk-and-prevention/breast-cancer-risk-factors.html

[41] Colditz GA, Bohlke K. Priorities for the primary prevention of breast cancer. CA: A Cancer Journal for Clinicians. 2014;**64**(3):186-194. DOI: 10.3322/caac.21225

[42] Saslow D, Boetes C, Burke W, Harms S, Leach MO, Lehman CD, et al. American Cancer Society breast cancer advisory group. American Cancer Society guidelines for breast screening with MRI as an adjunct to mammography. CA: A Cancer Journal for Clinicians. 2007;**57**(2):75-89. DOI: 10.3322/canjclin.57.2.75

[43] Waks AG, Winer EP. Breast cancer treatment: A review. Journal of the American Medical Association. 2019;**321**(3):288-300. DOI: 10.1001/jama.2018.19323

[44] Perou CM, Sørlie T, Eisen MB, van de Rijn M, Jeffrey SS, Rees CA, et al. Molecular portraits of human breast tumours. Nature. 2000;**406**(6797):747-752. DOI: 10.1038/35021093

[45] Curigliano G, Burstein HJ, Winer EP, Gnant M, Dubsky P, Loibl S, et al. St. Gallen international expert consensus on the primary therapy of early breast cancer 2017. Annals of Oncology. 2017;**28**(8):1700-1712. DOI: 10.1093/annonc/mdx308

[46] Lehmann BD, Bauer JA, Chen X, Sanders ME, Chakravarthy AB, Shyr Y, et al. Identification of human triple-negative breast cancer subtypes and preclinical models for selection of targeted therapies. The Journal of Clinical Investigation. 2011;**121**(7):2750-2767. DOI: 10.1172/JCI45014

[47] Martini R, Delpe P, Chu TR, Arora K, Lord B, Verma A, et al. African ancestry-associated gene expression profiles in triple-negative breast cancer underlie altered tumor biology and clinical outcome in women of African descent. Cancer Discovery. 2022;**12**(11):2530-2551. DOI: 10.1158/2159-8290.CD-22-0138

[48] Reid S, Fan R, Venton L, Weidner A, Tezak A, Roberson ML, et al. West African genetic ancestry and breast cancer outcomes among black women. JAMA Network Open. 2024;**7**(12):e2449798. DOI: 10.1001/jamanetworkopen.2024.49798

[49] Slamon DJ, Leyland-Jones B, Shak S, Fuchs H, Paton V, Bajamonde A, et al. Use of chemotherapy plus a monoclonal antibody against HER2 for metastatic breast cancer that overexpresses HER2. The New England Journal of Medicine. 2001;**344**(11):783-792. DOI: 10.1056/NEJM200103153441101

[50] Uygur MM, Gümüş M. The utility of serum tumor markers CEA and CA 15-3 for breast cancer prognosis and their association with clinicopathological parameters. Cancer Treatment and Research Communications. 2021;**28**:100402. DOI: 10.1016/j.ctarc.2021.100402

[51] Shao Y, Sun X, He Y, Liu C, Liu H. Elevated levels of serum tumor markers CEA and CA15-3 are prognostic parameters for different molecular subtypes of breast cancer. PLoS One. 2015;**10**(7):e0133830. DOI: 10.1371/journal.pone.0133830

[52] Rack B, Jückstock J, Trapp E, Weissenbacher T, Alunni-Fabbroni M, Schramm A, et al. SUCCESS study group. CA27.29 as a tumour marker for risk evaluation and therapy monitoring in primary breast cancer patients. Tumour Biology. 2016;**37**(10):13769-13775. DOI: 10.1007/s13277-016-5171-2

[53] Li S, Silvestri V, Leslie G, Rebbeck TR, Neuhausen SL, Hopper JL, et al. Cancer risks associated with BRCA1 and BRCA2 pathogenic variants. Journal of Clinical Oncology. 2022;**40**(14):1529-1541. DOI: 10.1200/JCO.21.02112

[54] Győrffy B, Hatzis C, Sanft T, Hofstatter E, Aktas B, Pusztai L. Multigene prognostic tests in breast cancer: Past, present, future. Breast Cancer Research. 2015;**17**(1):11. DOI: 10.1186/s13058-015-0514-2

[55] Duffy MJ, Harbeck N, Nap M, Molina R, Nicolini A, Senkus E, et al. Clinical use of biomarkers in breast cancer: Updated guidelines from the

European group on tumor markers (EGTM). European Journal of Cancer. 2017;**75**:284-298. DOI: 10.1016/j.ejca.2017.01.017

[56] Harbeck N, Kates RE, Look MP, Meijer-Van Gelder ME, Klijn JG, Krüger A, et al. Enhanced benefit from adjuvant chemotherapy in breast cancer patients classified high-risk according to urokinase-type plasminogen activator (uPA) and plasminogen activator inhibitor type 1 (n = 3424). Cancer Research. 2002;**62**(16):4617-4622

[57] Jacobs VR, Kates RE, Kantelhardt E, Vetter M, Wuerstlein R, Fischer T, et al. Health economic impact of risk group selection according to ASCO-recommended biomarkers uPA/PAI-1 in node-negative primary breast cancer. Breast Cancer Research and Treatment. 2013;**138**(3):839-850. DOI: 10.1007/s10549-013-2496-z

[58] Urbaniak C, Gloor GB, Brackstone M, Scott L, Tangney M, Reid G. The microbiota of breast tissue and its association with breast cancer. Applied and Environmental Microbiology. 2016;**82**(16):5039-5048. DOI: 10.1128/AEM.01235-16

[59] Hanahan D. Hallmarks of cancer: New dimensions. Cancer Discovery. 2022;**12**(1):31-46. DOI: 10.1158/2159-8290.CD-21-1059

[60] Zhang Y, Wang Y, Zhang B, Li P, Zhao Y. Methods and biomarkers for early detection, prediction, and diagnosis of colorectal cancer. Biomedicine and Pharmacotherapy. 2023;**163**:114786

[61] Song L, Jia J, Peng X, Xiao W, Li Y. The performance of the SEPT9 gene methylation assay and a comparison with other CRC screening tests: A meta-analysis. Scientific Reports. 2017;7:3032. DOI: 10.1038/s41598-017-03307-6

[62] Lech G. Colorectal cancer tumour markers and biomarkers: Recent therapeutic advances. World Journal of Gastroenterology. 2016;**22**(5):1745. DOI: 10.3748/wjg.v22.i5.1745

[63] Dienstmann R, Vermeulen L, Guinney J, Kopetz S, Tejpar S, Tabernero J. Consensus molecular subtypes and the evolution of precision medicine in colorectal cancer. Nature Reviews. Cancer. 2017;**17**(2):79-92. DOI: 10.1038/nrc.2016.126

[64] Fan A, Wang B, Wang X, Nie Y, Fan D, Zhao X, et al. Immunotherapy in colorectal cancer: Current achievements and future perspective. International Journal of Biological Sciences. 2021;**17**(14):3837-3849. DOI: 10.7150/ijbs.63543

[65] Keum N, Giovannucci E. Global burden of colorectal cancer: Emerging trends, risk factors and prevention strategies. Nature Reviews. Gastroenterology and Hepatology. 2019;**16**(12):713-732. DOI: 10.1038/s41575-019-0189-8

[66] Zhu G, Pei L, Xia H, Tang Q, Bi F. Role of oncogenic KRAS in the prognosis, diagnosis and treatment of colorectal cancer. Molecular Cancer. 2021;**20**(1):143. DOI: 10.1186/s12943-021-01441-4

[67] Sekhoacha M, Riet K, Motloung P, Gumenku L, Adegoke A, Mashele S. Prostate cancer review: Genetics, diagnosis, treatment options, and alternative approaches. Molecules. 2022;**27**(17):5730. DOI: 10.3390/molecules27175730

[68] Ilic D, Neuberger MM, Djulbegovic M, Dahm P. Screening for prostate cancer. Cochrane Database of Systematic Reviews. 2013;**2013**(1):CD004720. DOI: 10.1002/14651858.CD004720.pub3

[69] Rawla P. Epidemiology of prostate cancer. World Journal of Oncology. 2019;**10**(2):63-89. DOI: 10.14740/wjon1191

[70] Ebot EM, Gerke T, Labbé DP, Sinnott JA, Zadra G, Rider JR, et al. Gene expression profiling of prostate tissue identifies chromatin regulation as a potential link between obesity and lethal prostate cancer. Cancer. 2017;**123**(21):4130-4138. DOI: 10.1002/cncr.30831

[71] Udager AM, Tomlins SA. Molecular biomarkers in the clinical management of prostate cancer. Cold Spring Harbor Perspectives in Medicine. 2018;**8**(11):a030601. DOI: 10.1101/cshperspect.a030601

[72] Hamdy FC, Donovan JL, Lane JA, Mason M, Metcalfe C, Holding P, et al. ProtecT study group. 10-year outcomes after monitoring, surgery, or radiotherapy for localized prostate cancer. The New England Journal of Medicine. 2016;**375**(15):1415-1424. DOI: 10.1056/NEJMoa1606220

[73] Nyberg T, Frost D, Barrowdale D, Evans DG, Bancroft E, Adlard J, et al. Prostate cancer risks for male BRCA1 and BRCA2 mutation carriers: A prospective cohort study. European Urology. 2020;**77**(1):24-35. DOI: 10.1016/j.eururo.2019.08.025

[74] Jerónimo C, Henrique R. Epigenetic biomarkers in urological tumors: A systematic review. Cancer Letters. 2014;**342**(2):264-274. DOI: 10.1016/j.canlet.2011.12.026

[75] Tomlins SA, Rhodes DR, Perner S, Dhanasekaran SM, Mehra R, Sun XW, et al. Recurrent fusion of TMPRSS2 and ETS transcription factor genes in prostate cancer. Science. 2005;**310**(5748):644-648. DOI: 10.1126/science.1117679

[76] Parekh DJ, Punnen S, Sjoberg DD, Asroff SW, Bailen JL, Cochran JS, et al. A multi-institutional prospective trial in the USA confirms that the 4Kscore accurately identifies men with high-grade prostate cancer. European Urology. 2015;**68**(3):464-470. DOI: 10.1016/j.eururo.2014.10.021

[77] Loeb S, Sanda MG, Broyles DL, Shin SS, Bangma CH, Wei JT, et al. The prostate health index selectively identifies clinically significant prostate cancer. The Journal of Urology. 2015;**193**(4):1163-1169. DOI: 10.1016/j.juro.2014.10.121

[78] Borque-Fernando Á, Rubio-Briones J, Esteban LM, Dong Y, Calatrava A, Gómez-Ferrer Á, et al. Role of the 4Kscore test as a predictor of reclassification in prostate cancer active surveillance. Prostate Cancer and Prostatic Diseases. 2019;**22**(1):84-90. DOI: 10.1038/s41391-018-0074-5

[79] Marks LS, Fradet Y, Deras IL, Blase A, Mathis J, Aubin SM, et al. PCA3 molecular urine assay for prostate cancer in men undergoing repeat biopsy. Urology. 2007;**69**(3):532-535. DOI: 10.1016/j.urology.2006.12.014

[80] Xu J, Zheng SL, Komiya A, Mychaleckyj JC, Isaacs SD, Hu JJ, et al. Germline mutations and sequence variants of the macrophage scavenger receptor 1 gene are associated with prostate cancer risk. Nature Genetics. 2002;**32**(2):321-325. DOI: 10.1038/ng994

[81] Ewing CM, Ray AM, Lange EM, Zuhlke KA, Robbins CM, Tembe WD, et al. Germline mutations in HOXB13 and prostate-cancer risk. The New England Journal of Medicine. 2012;**366**(2):141-149. DOI: 10.1056/NEJMoa1110000

[82] Braun AE, Chan JM, Neuhaus J, Cowan JE, Kenfield SA, Van Blarigan EL,

et al. The impact of genomic biomarkers on a clinical risk prediction model for upgrading/upstaging among men with favorable-risk prostate cancer. Cancer. 2024;**130**(10):1766-1772. DOI: 10.1002/cncr.35215

[83] Partin AW, Van Neste L, Klein EA, Marks LS, Gee JR, Troyer DA, et al. Clinical validation of an epigenetic assay to predict negative histopathological results in repeat prostate biopsies. The Journal of Urology. 2014;**192**(4):1081-1087. DOI: 10.1016/j.juro.2014.04.013

[84] Petrillo A, Smyth EC. Biomarkers for precision treatment in gastric cancer. Visceral Medicine. 2020;**36**(5):364-372. DOI: 10.1159/000511053

[85] Matsuoka T, Yashiro M. Novel biomarkers for early detection of gastric cancer. World Journal of Gastroenterology. 2023;**29**(17):2515-2533. DOI: 10.3748/wjg.v29.i17.2515

[86] Laurén P. The two histological main types of gastric carcinoma: Diffuse and so-called intestinal-type carcinoma. Acta Pathologica et Microbiologica Scandinavica. 1965;**64**(1):31-49. DOI: 10.1111/apm.1965.64.1.31

[87] The Cancer Genome Atlas Research Network. Comprehensive molecular characterization of gastric adenocarcinoma. Nature. 2014;**513**(7517):202-209. DOI: 10.1038/nature13480

[88] Röcken C. Predictive biomarkers in gastric cancer. Journal of Cancer Research and Clinical Oncology. 2022;**148**(10):2535-2551. DOI: 10.1007/s00432-022-04192-1

[89] Polom K, Marrelli D, Smyth EC, Voglino C, Roviello G, Pascale V, et al. The role of microsatellite instability in positive margin gastric cancer patients. Surgical Innovation. 2018;**25**(2):99-104. DOI: 10.1177/1553350617751461

[90] Wang K, Yuen ST, Xu J, Lee SP, Yan HHN, Shi ST, et al. Whole-genome sequencing and comprehensive molecular profiling identify new driver mutations in gastric cancer. Nature Genetics. 2014;**46**(6):573-582. DOI: 10.1038/ng.2983

[91] Zang ZJ, Cutcutache I, Poon SL, Zhang SL, McPherson JR, Tao J, et al. Exome sequencing of gastric adenocarcinoma identifies recurrent somatic mutations in cell adhesion and chromatin remodeling genes. Nature Genetics. 2012;**44**(5):570-574. DOI: 10.1038/ng.2246

[92] Matsuoka T, Yashiro M. Biomarkers of gastric cancer: Current topics and future perspective. World Journal of Gastroenterology. 2018;**24**(26):2818-2832. DOI: 10.3748/wjg.v24.i26.2818

[93] Obermeyer Z, Emanuel EJ. Predicting the future—Big data, machine learning, and clinical medicine. The New England Journal of Medicine. 2016;**375**(13):1216-1219. DOI: 10.1056/NEJMp1606181

[94] Sharma P, Hu-Lieskovan S, Wargo JA, Ribas A. Primary, adaptive, and acquired resistance to cancer immunotherapy. Cell. 2017;**168**(4):707-723. DOI: 10.1016/j.cell.2017.01.017

[95] Gao J, Shi W, Wang J, Guan C, Dong Q, Sheng J, et al. Research progress and applications of epigenetic biomarkers in cancer. Frontiers in Pharmacology. 2024;**15**:1308309. DOI: 10.3389/fphar.2024.1308309

[96] Poste G, Compton CC, Barker AD. Biomarkers in cancer: The promise of personalized medicine. Nature Reviews. Cancer. 2021;**21**(3):131-142. DOI: 10.1038/s41568-020-00326-0

Chapter 5

A Practical Guide to Establishing a Molecular-Based Point-of-Care Testing Network for Chlamydia

Mark Shephard, Susan Matthews, Kelly Andrewartha, Gabi Hewer, Kirsty Smith, Louise Causer and Rebecca Guy

Abstract

This chapter provides a 'how to guide' to set up and manage a molecular-based point-of-care (POC) testing network to detect *Chlamydia trachomatis* (Chlamydia) in populations experiencing high burden of infection and sequelae as well as barriers to accessing routine laboratory services. The chapter outlines the experience of the Australian-based *Test, Treat and Go* (TTANGO) program which, to the authors' knowledge, represents the largest decentralised POC testing network for chlamydia (as well as gonorrhoea and trichomoniasis) in the primary care sector globally. The chapter provides an overview of the program's evolution from a randomised controlled trial through implementation, translation, and scale-up phases to a now national routine program with associated testing rebates. The chapter will examine the governance, training and quality management, and connectivity processes that underpin the TTANGO network and describe the clinical, cultural, operational and economic effectiveness of the network. Collectively, these elements provide a template for translation to low- and middle-income countries (LMIC) where *Chlamydia trachomatis* remains a significant contemporary health problem.

Keywords: point-of-care testing, primary care, chlamydia, sexually transmitted infections, decentralised

1. Introduction

1.1 Defining the clinical problem

Chlamydia is a very common sexually transmitted infection (STI) that is caused by the bacterium *Chlamydia trachomatis* (CT) and transmitted by unprotected sexual activity. Chlamydia remains a major contemporary health problem globally, with more than 128.5 million new cases of this infection being reported in adults aged between 15 and 49 years during 2020 [1, 2]. Collectively, chlamydia, as well as other related pathogens *Neisseria gonorrhoeae* (gonorrhoea, NG), *Trichomonas vaginalis* (trichomoniasis, TV), and *Treponema pallidum* (syphilis, TP), accounted for more than one million new infections every day during 2020 [3]. Left untreated or undetected, chlamydia can have serious consequences, mainly in women, with pelvic inflammatory disease (PID) as well as tubal infertility and ectopic pregnancy being critical examples of onward sequelae [4, 5].

In Australia, young First Nations people experience among the highest rates of chlamydia (as well as gonorrhoea and trichomoniasis) in the world, with one third of all First Nations adults aged between 16 and 29 years testing positive for one or more of these infections during the period 2009–2011 [6]. The magnitude of the problem is exacerbated by a range of complex and interwoven social, cultural, and economic determinants of health and geographic factors including high mobility of remote populations; as well as lack of access to culturally appropriate health services, including pathology testing.

Fortunately, confirmed cases of chlamydia are readily treatable and curable, with azithromycin or doxycycline being the drugs of choice most widely used for the treatment of uncomplicated genital chlamydia infections [7].

1.2 Diagnostic capacity and the role of POC testing

In many LMIC, syndromic management is the first line of treatment for chlamydia and related infections, but this approach can lead to missed diagnoses if patients are asymptomatic or overtreatment (potentially with the wrong antibiotic) when the causative agent is not identified.

Clearly, the need for the early detection of chlamydia through regular pathology testing is the key to accurately identifying both asymptomatic and symptomatic infections and assisting in breaking the cycle of onward (or vertical) transmission. While access to pathology laboratories in urban settings is generally readily available, the use of laboratory testing for diagnosis in rural and remote regions is more problematic, and (from the Australian experience) uptake of testing has been relatively low [8]. Also, the turnaround time for laboratory results on samples collected from rural and remote communities can often be between 1 and 2 weeks, but importantly, the time for patient follow-up and treatment can be even longer, up to several weeks [9].

Molecular-based point-of-care (POC) pathology testing for STIs such as chlamydia has the potential to be a 'game changer', particularly in the rural and remote context, as the test can be conducted during the patient consultation with the result available within a significantly shorter time frame (i.e., within hours) and facilitate more rapid initiation of curative treatment and partner notification.

Chronologically, POC testing was seeded in the global primary care setting during the late 1990s/early 2000s through chronic disease applications (notably diabetes and renal and heart disease) and then in acute care settings (for tests such as electrolytes, blood gases, and cardiac troponin) [10]. Historically, the uptake of POC testing for infectious disease up to the early-2010s was limited to immunochromatographic lateral flow technologies which suffered from poor analytical performance, notably poor sensitivity [7]. However, the advent of molecular-based technologies (namely, nucleic acid amplification tests which detect DNA or RNA from infectious agents) has completely transformed this field through substantial improvements in simplified test process, closed cartridge systems and diagnostic accuracy, with development and application of a wide test menu for POC testing for infectious disease now outstripping those of chronic and acute modalities.

However, while the market for POC testing for infectious disease has grown exponentially in combination with an increased demand for public health research impact, there is a critical need to consider how to systematically and sustainably integrate POC testing in this field. Importantly, foundational medical science implementation and scale-up strategies that prioritise patient safety and optimise diagnostic accuracy are essential in enabling the desired clinical and public health benefits from such disruptive technology [10, 11].

This chapter draws on the Australian experience and lessons learned from field application of POC testing across chronic, acute, and infectious diseases over the past 25 years to provide a 'how to guide' to set up and manage a molecular-based point-of-care (POC) testing network to detect *Chlamydia trachomatis* (Chlamydia) infection in at-risk rural, remote, and/or disadvantaged communities [10–12].

2. An optimised program logic framework for the implementation and management of a POC testing network: From concept to public health impact

The key to the development of sustainable and impactful POC testing is a systematic and stepwise program logic model to its integration in primary care. The steps involved in this process are outlined in **Figure 1**.

Firstly, there must be an identified and defined clinical need to justify the introduction and establishment of a POC testing service. A clinical needs assessment should be undertaken in consultation with appropriate multidisciplinary clinical teams and tailored to meet local, jurisdictional, or national needs. The proposed POC testing solution will be dependent on factors such as population size, age structure, ethnicity and culture, geographic location and accessibility or otherwise to a pathology laboratory service, and availability and expertise of local health service staff [13].

There must be universal acceptance and recognition from stakeholders in their decision to adopt this technology that POC testing is a medical science discipline. The successful translation of POC testing from the laboratory to the field is dependent on adherence to and adaptation of core laboratory principles and standard good

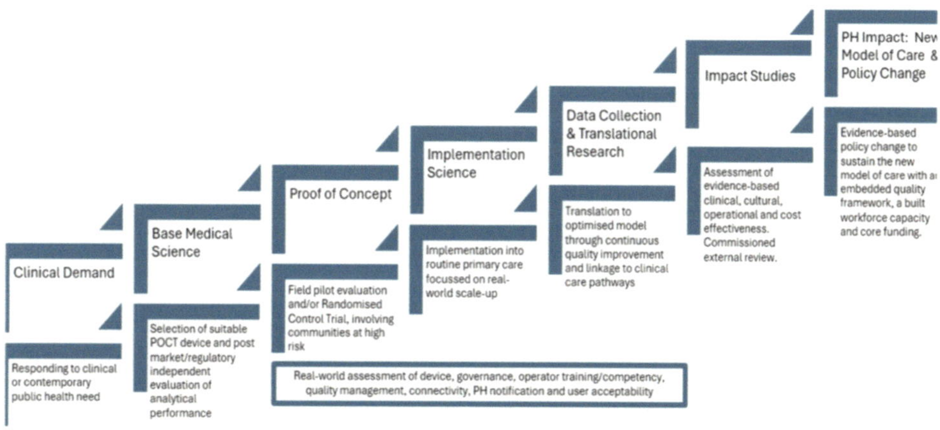

Figure 1.
The systematic and stepwise building of a sustainable and impactful POC testing model © Matthews S and Shephard M, 2024.

laboratory practices (notably relating to device selection, training of non-laboratory health professionals, analytical method and surveillance of analytical quality, and minimisation of preanalytical and postanalytical sources of error) which mitigate patient harm.

In today's global market, there are often multiple devices available that can potentially perform the required POC tests. It is important to critically review the manufacturer's claims, existing regulatory approvals, independent published literature available on these devices or, as a minimum, consult with professional colleagues, notably pathologists and medical scientists, who have had experience with result interpretation and safe practice with the device(s) concerned. As a guiding principle, a POC testing device should be able to achieve at least equivalent analytical performance for the required tests compared to the corresponding laboratory device when used for the same clinical purpose.

Critically, the performance of devices must be verified independently in a 'proof of concept' phase; this applies not only to an assessment of the analytical quality of the device but also to non-analytical factors such as ease of specimen collection; user friendliness/stakeholder acceptability; complexity of use, including the number of manual steps involved; physical footprint within the health service (including ancillary needs for storage of testing reagents and requirements for AC or battery power); environmental friendliness and real-time connectivity (particularly in the face of poor or non-existent internet availability); and a cost-benefit analysis of introducing the device (investigating the balance between affordability, accessibility, and diagnostic accuracy, as well as covering both fixed and variable costs) [14].

Independent evaluation of the device should be undertaken either at/with the support of the local pathology laboratory and then, ideally, at the intended site of field use by the (trained) operators who would be conducting tests in routine practice at their service. Field evaluation can occur, for example, as a pilot study or as part of a randomised controlled trial (across a small number of targeted sites that are known to service communities with a high burden of disease) to allow comparison to the usual standard of care.

The next stepwise phases involve broader implementation of the program to reach more targeted sites with high disease prevalence and to systematically scale up the program to reach the point where POC testing becomes part of routine practice.

In these implementation/translational phases, the following core regulatory elements should be embedded into the system:

- Establishing appropriate governance of the network, including both clinical, scientific, and cultural governance
- Training of POC testing operators including initial and ongoing assessment of their competency
- Continuous surveillance of analytical quality, through application of standard laboratory practices such as quality control (QC) and external quality assurance (EQA) testing
- Intensive scientific and technical support for trained operators (including device troubleshooting and corrective actions, as well as logistic support for delivery of consumables and quality testing materials)

- Connectivity (the electronic capture of patient results and their transference to a patient medical record, to public health authorities for surveillance and to the program for monitoring implementation).

All these elements should be subjected to stakeholder evaluation, internal quality auditing processes, and actioning of opportunities for process improvement to ensure continuous quality improvement (CQI) practices and optimisation of the routine model.

Ideally, at this point, POC testing should also be integrated into relevant clinical pathways for patient care and management. Adherence to jurisdictional or national guidelines, requirements, or standards for POC testing should also be followed.

It should be noted that there are opportunities for stakeholder engagement, co-design and both quantitative and qualitative research to be conducted along the spectrum of activities described thus far, with research findings relating to the analytical performance in the field and laboratory, as well as stakeholder acceptability being examples of key questions to be answered at this point.

However, once the primary care model is fully operational and scaled, then it is possible to develop specific research activities to assess the clinical, cultural, operational, and economic impacts of introducing this POC testing service for its intended purpose [15]. For infectious diseases, clinical benefits usually focus on measures such as increased testing uptake, earlier detection of disease, reduction in time to initiate treatment, and days of infections averted. Cultural benefits are important when the work supports rural and remote indigenous health services and communities; here, patient satisfaction with the process of POC testing and reduction in loss to follow-up are key outcome measures. Operational benefits focusing on POC testing operator and medical practitioner satisfaction are important to assess, with the increased sense of responsibility and empowerment for operators and immediacy of clinical decision making for doctors being important considerations. Until the past decade, cost effectiveness had not been researched well in POC testing studies, but now, this measure has become increasingly important as governments seek an evidence-base of measurable cost benefits in determining whether to fund POC testing activities and their associated return on investment [16, 17].

Finally, when all steps have been scientifically and robustly implemented, the larger-scale public health impacts of the POC testing model may be realised; these may relate to the new model of care bringing about evidence-based policy change; building a large and resilient workforce capacity; or, in the specific case of infectious diseases, averting significant numbers of infectious days for a jurisdiction or nation, complementing national diagnostic testing frameworks (as seen in COVID-19) and providing an evidence-base for inclusion within pathology testing rebating schemes (such as described below).

Timewise, the evolution of a POC testing model from a medical science concept to broad impact may take a decade or more, but with all elements systematically implemented, the model is most likely to be well accepted, deliver high analytical quality, and minimise patient risk and thus be sustainable.

3. Application of this stepwise template to POC testing for chlamydia: The Australian experience

In Australia, the Flinders University International Centre for Point-of-Care Testing (ICPOCT) and the Kirby Institute, University of New South Wales, jointly manage several POC testing networks for infectious diseases on behalf of the Australian Government's Department of Health and Aged Care [11]. The longest standing network, now of more than a decade's duration, is the *Test, Treat ANd GO* (TTANGO) program which, to our knowledge, represents the largest decentralised molecular-based POC testing network for chlamydia (as well as gonorrhoea and trichomoniasis) in the primary care sector globally.

Following the stepwise template outlined above, we will now describe the evolution of the TTANGO network from concept to public health impact.

3.1 Responding to clinical need

The clinical need for a POC testing program to detect chlamydia (and gonorrhoea) resulted from a disproportionately high burden of these STIs in young adults living in remote First Nations communities and a call to action from clinicians. The aim of introducing POC testing was to detect new cases of these infections, thereby enabling faster initiation of curative treatment, reducing the risk of sequelae and onward transmission to partners, and decreasing overall disease prevalence in the community.

3.2 Evaluation of new molecular-based POC testing technology

The GeneXpert® testing system (Cepheid, USA) was first introduced into Australia in 2013. The GeneXpert measures chlamydia and gonorrhoea on a single test cartridge using molecular based, nucleic acid amplification [NAAT] technology – detecting a single DNA target for chlamydia and dual DNA targets (NG2 and NG4) for gonorrhoea, and with a result turnaround time of 90 minutes. The GeneXpert system comprises a laptop required to drive the testing process, a modular GeneXpert device (four-module being the preferred configuration for TTANGO services), and closed testing cartridges for the simultaneous dual measurement of CT and NG.

The device underwent two initial evaluations—one in the laboratory setting and one in the primary care environment [18, 19].

The laboratory evaluation conducted GeneXpert POC tests on 372 characterised CT (or NG) bacterial strains and concluded the Xpert CT/NG testing cartridge was highly sensitive and specific for these infectious agents [18].

Just under 2500 (2486) self-collected urine or lower vaginal swabs were tested by both the GeneXpert POC test on-site in the field and parallel NAAT-based laboratory tests. The overall concordance for chlamydia was 99.4% (95% confidence intervals [CI] 99.1–99.7%) with a positive concordance of 98.6% (CI 95.9–99.7%) and negative concordance of 99.5% (CI 99.1–99.8%) (POC testing for NG demonstrated similar overall concordance of 99.9% compared to parallel laboratory testing) [19].

3.3 Proof of concept: The TTANGO trial (2013–2015)

The field evaluation of the CT/NG POC test was conducted as part of a cluster-randomised crossover trial called the TTANGO Trial. The TTANGO Trial, undertaken from 2013 to 2015, represented the first phase in the evolution of the (now national) TTANGO Program and the world-first use of molecular-based POC technology for STI in a primary care setting (outside the laboratory environment). The three-year TTANGO Trial was undertaken in 12 remote Aboriginal health services, which were spread across three Australian states (Western Australia, South Australia and

Queensland) and encompassed outer regional, remote or very remote locations. These services all met the following inclusion criteria: their health service conducted more than 150 CT/NG tests annually on young adults aged between 16 and 29 years and had a positivity rate for either CT or NG of 10% of higher. Services were randomised equally to either standard care with laboratory testing for 12 months (control group) followed by the additional availability of POC testing for the next 12 months (intervention group) or the reverse modality [19].

In addition to the excellent analytical performance observed during the trial (as described above), clinical effectiveness (time-to-treat) studies identified that 60% of the 455 patients who tested positive for CT/NG in the intervention group were treated in ≤2 days compared to 30% of the 405 patients who were diagnosed as positive using laboratory testing; while 76% of those patients in the intervention group were treated in ≤7 days compared to 47% when laboratory testing was used for diagnosis [20].

POC testing operators trained during the trial participated in in-depth interviews and questionnaires to assess their level of acceptability with the new technology. Overall, they reported the GeneXpert was user-friendly and useful in the primary care setting, while POC testing had improved STI management through more timely and targeted treatment, earlier commencement of partner notification and reduced time and effort associated with patient recall [7, 21]. From the patient perspective, the perceived usefulness of the POC technology centred on the following aspects: POC testing almost entirely eliminated the need for patient recall associated with previous laboratory-based testing; POC testing reduced the time between sample collection and delivery of treatment, an important consideration when acknowledging the significant population mobility in remote communities; and POC testing heightened awareness of STIs among community members as well as creating an opportunity for broader health education (particularly while the patient was waiting in the clinic for their test result) [21].

3.4 Implementation and scale-up phase (TTANGO2 and TTANGO3) (2016–2024)

Following the success of the randomised controlled trial, the Australian Government funded the scale-up of molecular-based STI POC testing through (i) a translational research program (called TTANGO2) which operated from 2016 to 2019 and then (ii) the routine implementation of the program (TTANGO3) from 2020 to 2024. As part of the scale-up process, molecular-based POC testing for TV on the GeneXpert was added to the TTANGO2 STI panel in April 2018, following regulatory approval of this test by the Australian Therapeutic Goods Administration (TGA) and independent evaluation of the test performance by the TTANGO study organisers [22].

Scale-up has continued to the present day, with the number of enrolled health services increasing to 31 by 2019, 58 by 2022, and 76, as of August 2024, with the TTANGO program now having a reach across all mainland Australian states and the Northern Territory (**Figures 2** and **3**). The jurisdictional breakdown of enrolled services is as follows: Western Australia 25, Northern Territory 17, Queensland 15, South Australia 10, New South Wales 6, and Victoria 3.

The guidelines for inclusion as a participating health service in the current program include being in a community classified as regional, remote or very remote, where the community prevalence of two STIs (CT, NG, or TV) in 15–29-year-olds is 10% or higher, and where the health service must service predominantly Aboriginal or Torres Strait Islander people (>50%).

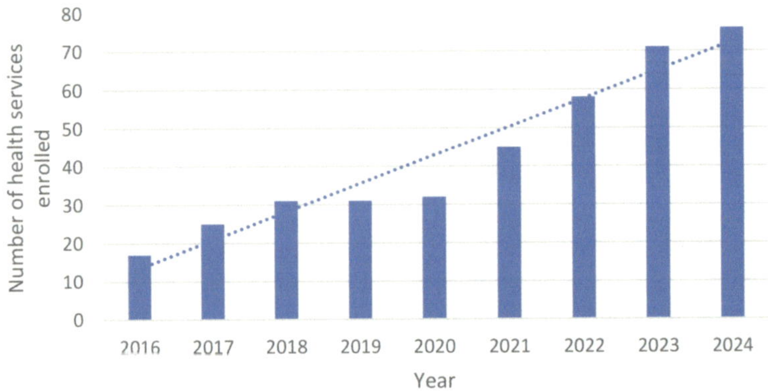

Figure 2.
Cumulative increase in total enrolments within TTANGO (2016–2024).

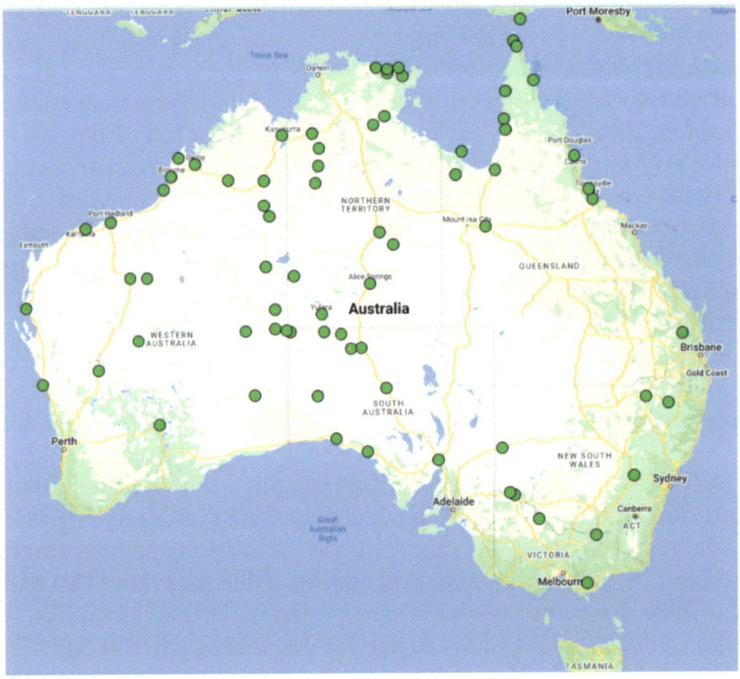

Figure 3.
Location of services enrolled in TTANGO Program, August 2024.

Core elements embedded in the routine operational model include the following:

3.4.1 Governance

During TTANGO2, the governance structure included an investigator group, an executive (management) committee, and an operational group. The executive (management) committee comprised senior TTANGO researchers from the lead academic institutions as well as a representative from the state/territory governments and the jurisdictional First Nations health bodies involved. The management committee oversaw the TTANGO operational team who were responsible for the day-to-day management, delivery and logistics of the program and who collaborated with a range of partners including those from industry and suppliers of quality materials. As a complementary CQI measure, a TTANGO Aboriginal and Torres Strait Islander Reference Group (comprising at least one Aboriginal and/or Torres Strait Islander Health Worker/Practitioner from each State/Territory who was also an active POC testing operator in the program) was established in 2018. The Reference Group advised on cultural safety (notably in relation to training resource development and promotional resources) and acted as cultural ambassadors for the program; this latter group was suspended during the COVID-19 pandemic but has resumed operation in 2024 known as the First Nations POC Testing Leaders Group (**Figure 4**).

3.4.2 Training and competency assessment of POC testing operators

A series of flexible training resources were developed for the program including a hard copy manual, laminated poster sets comprising step-by-step guides for the conduct of patient and quality testing practices, instructional videos, and access to an on-line version of these resources via a password-protected area on the program's website (www.ttango.com.au).

In terms of training delivery, options include on-site face-to-face training (at both individual services and regional training sessions) as well as web-based tele- or video-conference platforms (including GoToMeeting, TEAMS, and Webex—desktop sharing programs that allow users to interact with trainers online in real-time via the internet). Since early 2024, a new Learning Management System (LMS) has been introduced as an alternative to in-person or videoconference training which continue to be available to health services. The LMS is an online (Moodle-based) platform where operators can undertake self-guided theoretical training and competency for the TTANGO program, as well as for other POC testing networks for infectious diseases managed by ICPOCT/Kirby (see later); LMS training is facilitated by a series of self-guided modules which include disease-specific modules applicable to individual programs such as TTANGO as well as generic POC testing modules which apply to the broader Flinders ICPOCT/Kirby suite of infectious disease POC testing networks and quality systems.

No matter which mode of training delivery is used, all GeneXpert operators are required to undertake both theoretical and practical competency assessments; the

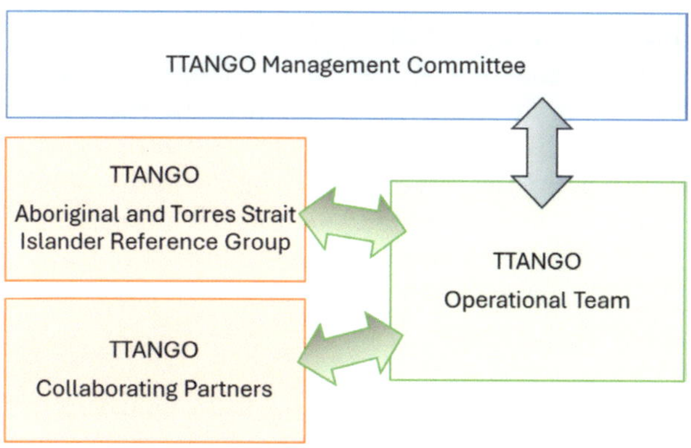

Figure 4.
Governance structure for the TTANGO routine operational program.

former involves completing a multiple-choice written assessment while the latter is assessed by performing practical tests on the GeneXpert using samples with a known infection load (previously specifically manufactured training samples, now QC samples). Unique operator logins used for GeneXpert testing and quality test result submission, and certificates of competency are issued for a period of 1 year to operators who successfully complete both the theoretical and practical components. Following expiry, operators must undergo a competency renewal process to be able to continue patient testing.

3.4.3 Quality management

To monitor the analytical quality of the GeneXpert devices in TTANGO, each health service is required to perform regular testing of quality control (QC) and external quality assurance (EQA) samples.

From 2016 to 2022, services tested one CT/NG positive QC swab sample (and one TV positive QC swab sample post 2018) each month on their GeneXpert. These samples were made in-house for the program [23]. Since March 2023, a commercial supplier (Microbix Biosystems Inc) has been contracted to provide both a positive and negative quality control swab material for the program. Operators enter their QC testing results online through the participant only area on the TTANGO website; here, immediate feedback on the accuracy of the result is available using a colour-coded action system which directs operators to appropriate QC actioning strategies (for discordant QC or test errors).

Health services are required to complete External Quality Assurance (EQA) testing using dry swab samples of varying infectious loads prepared specifically for the TTANGO program by the National Serology Reference Laboratory (NRL). From 2016 to 2020, there were two testing events comprising four swabs per event. From 2021 onwards, there were three testing events with five swabs to be tested per event. Each EQA swab has an expected result, which is unknown to the operator at the time of testing. Results are entered online via the TTANGO website and the TTANGO scientific team then prepare site-specific EQA reports which are issued to the operators who conducted the testing as well as health service managers/supervisors. Each report demonstrates how the services' GeneXpert results compare to the expected results and to other participating health services in a de-identified manner.

It should be noted that parallel laboratory testing has continued to be performed on each patient sample tested at the POC on the GeneXpert which has provided a further means of monitoring analytical quality and patient safety while also maintaining mandatory public health notifications for chlamydia (and gonorrhoea). Parallel laboratory testing will be phased out in November 2024 with the establishment of alternative notification pathways and changes to public health policy to recognise POC testing in the case definition for mandatory notifications of chlamydia (and gonorrhoea) cases.

3.4.4 Scientific and technical support

The TTANGO operational team provides a scientific help desk which operates during business hours (9 am to 5 pm) during the working week. The help desk offers support for issues relating to troubleshooting, technical issues, maintenance and logistics, as well as interpretation of QC results and EQA reports.

3.4.5 Connectivity

A tailored connectivity system was built for the TTANGO program to capture digital POC test results for CT/NG and TV electronically and deliver them to a range of end users for the purposes of clinical management; surveillance of analytical quality; program implementation; and public health surveillance through the mandatory notification of positive CT (and NG) results which are notifiable diseases within Australia. The notification process also extends to TV, which is a notifiable disease in the Northern Territory [24]. The connectivity system represented the first of its type in Australia that was established independent of laboratory pathology providers to support POC testing for infectious disease in remote primary health services.

3.5 Key findings and assessment of evidence-based outcomes

3.5.1 Uptake of POC testing (2016-present)

During the 7-year period between 2016 and 2022, 30,160 CT/NG (and 15,993 TV) POC tests were performed in the TTANGO Program (total 46,153 tests) [25]. The statistically significant upward trend in testing numbers observed during the first 4 years of the program was dampened during the subsequent period of April 2020 to December 2022 due to the influence of the COVID-19 pandemic when health professional resources were diverted away from mainstream care activities. As of August 2024, the total number of STI POC tests performed has now exceeded 55,000. Positivity rates for CT (and NG and TV) during the 2022–2024 period were approximately 10% (and 9 and 8.5%) respectively.

3.5.2 Training and competency assessment

From January 2016 to June 2024, 1243 health professionals attended a TTANGO GeneXpert training session; a total of 803 (56%) received face-to-face training and 402 (32%) attended training remotely via web-based online platforms. Face-to-face training was the main form of training delivery prior to the COVID-19 pandemic, while travel restrictions during the pandemic saw a shift towards online platforms post 2022 (**Figure 5**). Since the recent introduction of the LMS training option in 2024, 38 new operators have been trained using this modality.

Of the 1243 who undertook training, 1002 (81%) successfully completed the new operator competency assessment process.

From January 2016 to June 2024, a total of 1294 operator competencies were completed, comprising new operators (n = 1002 [77%]) and operators renewing their competency (n = 292 [23%]).

Nurses continue to be the main health professional group trained in TTANGO, representing 72% (719/1002) of new operators trained, while Aboriginal Health Workers/Practitioners made up 21% (206/1002) of the new operator pool. A breakdown of new operator competencies by profession and year is shown in **Figure 6**.

3.5.3 Analytical quality

From 2016 to 2022, the concordance between GeneXpert POC patient testing and parallel laboratory NAAT testing was 99.0% (4071/4111) for CT (and 99.3% for NG and 98.9% for TV) [25]. Among the very low number of discordant results, there was

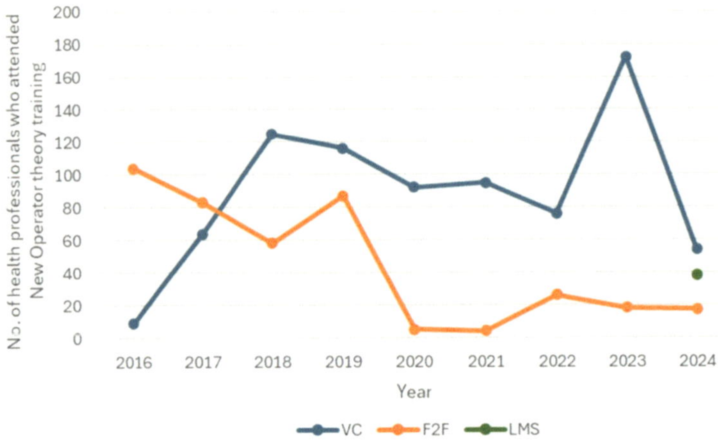

Figure 5.
New operator training attendance, by modality (Jan 2016–June 2024).

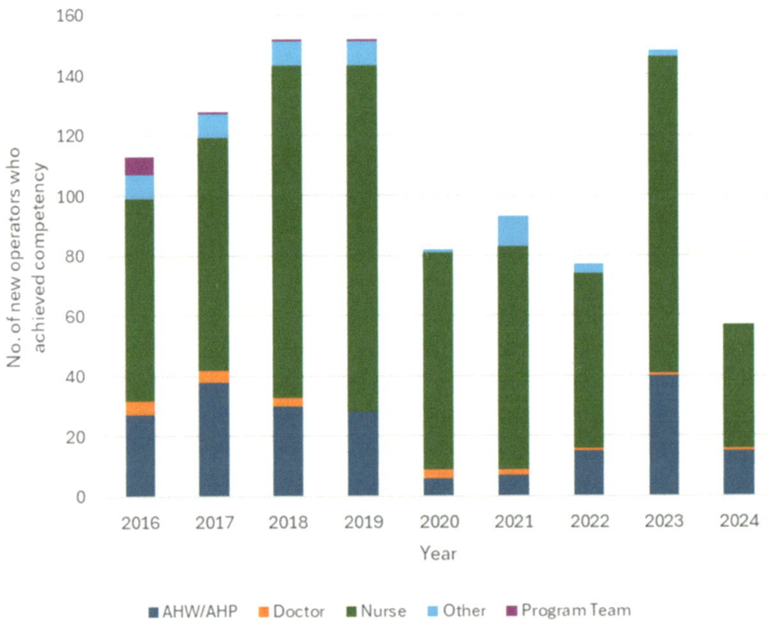

Figure 6.
New operator competency certifications, split by profession and year.

no specific pattern associated with either program sites or year of testing. The number of unsuccessful CT/NG tests (subcategorised as 'invalid', 'error', or 'no result') on the GeneXpert was 3.1% (which fell to 1.8% when samples were available for retesting).

Figure 7 summarises the results of QC testing conducted since the introduction of the commercial Microbix QC product in April 2023. In total, just over 1700 QC tests for CT were performed in the 12-month period from April 2023 to April 2024. Overall concordance with the expected result on just over 1600 valid QC tests was 97.0% (1558/1606), with concordance for the positive QC being 97.4% (795/816) and concordance for the negative QC 96.6% (763/790). The majority of the discordant results were attributed to transcription errors in reporting of results, which triggered retraining of operators. Rates of unsuccessful QC tests for CT were less than 6% (102/1708), most of which were due to an 'invalid' test result being reported (see footnote to **Figure 7**).

Table 1 summarises the results of EQA testing across the most recent three testing cycles conducted during 2023. There were 15 EQA samples tested, six that were positive for CT with varying infectious loads and nine negative samples for CT. In total, 571 (560 + 11) tests were performed during this one-year period. The overall concordance with the expected EQA result on the 560 valid tests was 97.3% (553/560), with concordance for the positive EQA samples being 96.9% (222/229) and concordance for the negative EQA 97.2% (322/331). Rates of unsuccessful QC tests for CT were less than 3% (11/571).

3.5.4 Clinical effectiveness

Consistent with the findings of the original TTANGO Trial, clinical effectiveness studies conducted during TTANGO from 2016 to 2019 showed that patients testing positive for CT and/or NG by POC testing were treated more rapidly than those undergoing laboratory testing [25]. The median time to treat following a positive CT and/or NG POC test was 1 day (interquartile range [IQR] 0–3) compared to 11 days for a positive laboratory test (IQR 0–65). A greater proportion of patients testing positive in the intervention period were treated compared to the control period across all time periods (≤2 days 37 versus 22%; and ≤ 7 days 48 versus 30%, respectively). Based on this difference in median time to treat, study researchers estimated that POC testing for CT (and NG and TV) averted 4930 (and 5620 and 7075) infectious days, during this four-year period [25].

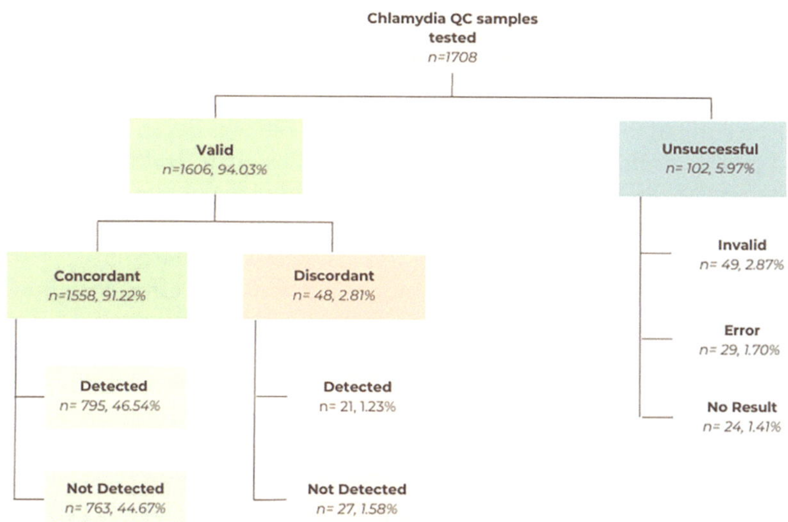

Figure 7.
QC testing performed in TTANGO post the introduction of dual testing samples since April 2023. Note: 'Invalid' tests can occur due to a multitude of operator, cartridge, and device-related issues, while 'error' and 'no result' usually reflect device-related or power-related issues.

Survey ID	Sample ID	Expected result	Submitted results		
			Not detected %(*n*)	**Detected** %(*n*)	**Unsuccessful** %(*n*)
Survey 1 2023-04-21	Sample A	Detected	*2.56% (1)*	*92.31% (36)*	*5.13% (2) [no result]*
	Sample B	Not detected	*94.87% (37)*	*5.13% (2)*	*0.0% (0)*
	Sample C	Not detected	*94.87% (37)*	*2.56% (1)*	*2.56% (1) [no result]*
	Sample D	Detected	*12.63% (1)*	*60.66% (37)*	*0.0% (0)*
	Sample E	Not detected	*89.47% (34)*	*5.26% (2)*	*5.26% (2) [no result]*
Survey 2 2023-07-19	Sample A	Detected	*0.0% (0)*	*100% (34)*	*0.0% (0)*
	Sample B	Not detected	*100% (35)*	*0.0% (0)*	*0.0% (0)*
	Sample C	Not detected	*100% (35)*	*0.0% (0)*	*0.0% (0)*
	Sample D	Not detected	*85.71% (30)*	*8.57% (3)*	*5.71% (2) [no result]*
	Sample E	Not detected	*100% (35)*	*0.0% (0)*	*0.0% (0)*
Survey 3 2023-10-18	Sample A	Not detected	*97.56% (40)*	*2.44% (1)*	*0.0% (0)*
	Sample B	Detected	*2.44% (1)*	*95.12% (39)*	*2.44% (1) [invalid]*
	Sample C	Detected	*4.88% (2)*	*92.68% (38)*	*2.44% (1) [invalid]*
	Sample D	Not detected	*97.56% (40)*	*0.0% (0)*	*2.44% (1) [invalid]*
	Sample E	Detected	*4.88% (2)*	*92.68% (38)*	*2.44% (1) [invalid]*

Boxes highlighted in green indicate the percentage (%) and number (n) of results which were concordant with the expected QA results; boxes in red indicate the percentage (%) and number (n) of results which were discordant with the expected QA result; boxes in yellow indicate the percentage (%) and number of results that were unsuccessful.

Table 1.
Summary of results from 3 EQA testing cycles during 2023.

3.5.5 Operational effectiveness

A follow-up acceptability study was conducted during the implementation phase of TTANGO2 to explore the facilitators and barriers to enable the optimised scale-up of STI POC testing in the remote First Nations sector [26]. In-depth interviews were conducted with 15 healthcare workers (nurses and Aboriginal Health Workers) and five managers from seven health services with a spread of geographic remoteness and varying STI POC testing rates. Acceptability of STI POC in TTANGO2 was high, due mainly to the self-efficacy (confidence and competence in the ability to perform the test and implement STI POC testing readily) and perceived effectiveness of the technology (the extent to which POC testing was perceived as likely to achieve its intended purpose/the effectiveness of the STI POC testing pathway versus laboratory testing and standard STI test-and-treat pathways). Patient reach (including strategies for patient engagement) was also considered an enabler of POC testing scale-up.

The main barrier to POC testing implementation was the high rate of turnover among staff working in the remote setting [26], which is an ongoing issue within remote health in Australia, in general. To try and increase the uptake of POC testing operator training, the TTANGO program has recently implemented an online learning platform to make the training more accessible to health service staff, particularly those on short-term contracts. The program team are also investigating alternative workforce models, including the possibility of training non-clinical staff to conduct

POC testing; this could include staff local to the community providing a more stable operator pool.

3.5.6 Cost effectiveness

A recent study evaluated the cost-effectiveness of using molecular POC testing for chlamydia, gonorrhoea and trichomoniasis compared to standard laboratory testing. Using a decision analytic model comparing the costs (mean cost per person tested) and outcomes (quality adjusted life year gain [QALY]) over a 10-year time horizon, the study found POC testing for these three infections was likely to be cost-effective in remote communities. The main drivers of reduced costs for molecular POC testing compared to laboratory testing were decreased staff time required for follow-up of patients for treatment and decreased incidence of hospitalisations for acute PID and other sequelae including ectopic pregnancy, as well as decreased incidence of preterm births and low birth weight babies. The one-way sensitivity analysis showed that the variables most likely to affect the incremental cost effectiveness ratio were the prevalence of STIs, the cost of the POC test, and health care attendance of women as a proportion of all attendees. In all sensitivity analyses POC testing remained either less costly or cost effective compared to laboratory testing and was under the threshold for public funding in Australia [27, 28].

4. Broad public health impact of the TTANGO STI POC testing program

The range of evidence-based outcome benefits demonstrated in TTANGO (reported above) has now led to broader public health impacts as well as policy change at the national government level.

During the recent global COVID-19 pandemic, the Australian Government invited the Kirby Institute and Flinders ICPOCT to develop a POC testing network to deliver molecular-based POC testing for SARS-CoV-2 using the GeneXpert in the most remote and vulnerable First Nations communities across the country; this so-named Aboriginal and Torres Strait Islander COVID-19 POC Testing network literally serviced those communities that were outside the reach of both urban and regional Australian laboratories. In setting up this emergency response network in early 2020, we were able to leverage the existing TTANGO program which already had established training, quality, and connectivity systems in place as well as a significant work-ready and skilled workforce who were competent in performing GeneXpert tests. The (then) 35 TTANGO services formed the first intake of sites in the COVID-19 network, which was supplemented by the addition of more than 60 further services that were provided with GeneXpert devices by the Australian Government. The Aboriginal and Torres Strait Islander COVID-19 POC Testing Program made a major contribution to Australia's public health response to the pandemic, averting between 23,000 and 122,000 SARS-Cov-2 infections and saving the Australian healthcare system between $337 Million and $1.8 Billion in health costs [11, 17, 29, 30].

In June 2022, the Aboriginal and Torres Strait Islander COVID-19 POC Testing Program transitioned to a new multiplex respiratory test panel which enabled SARS-CoV-2 as well as influenza A, influenza B, and respiratory syncytial virus (RSV) POC tests to be performed on a single cartridge. In early 2024, the TTANGO STI and Respiratory Infections networks merged to form the national First Nations Molecular POC Testing Program.

In its federal budget in May 2024, the Australian Government Department of Health and Aged Care announced a new Medicare rebate item for STI POC testing undertaken by remote and very remote health services (Modified Monash Model MM6 and MM7 [31]) in the First Nations Molecular POC Testing Program. The rebate, to commence in November 2024, includes funding to not only cover the cost of the consumables required for CT/NG and TV POC testing, but also a component to cover workforce capacity to perform the tests. Importantly, the rebate was contingent on eligible services continuing to participate in and demonstrate sound analytical performance for QC and EQA STI testing.

5. Discussion and concluding remarks

5.1 Comparison of TTANGO with other international POC testing programs for sexually transmitted infections

The TTANGO Program is unique in its scale (76 sites and 6 jurisdictions), geographic reach (rural and remote Australia), setting (primary health care, Aboriginal community controlled and government managed), strong Indigenous governance, networked connectivity (for program oversight, clinical management and notifiable disease reporting), operational implementation (in a non-laboratory environment), training and operational support (developed and delivered to cater to primary care clinician end-users), and, as of November 2024, sustained public funding.

In the United Kingdom, the Dean Street Express clinic has been offering molecular POC testing for STIs (chlamydia and gonorrhoea) as part of a rapid testing service for asymptomatic screening for several years [32]. While using the same GeneXpert technology as the TTANGO program and conducting high volumes of testing, this service is limited to one urban location in central London and is implemented through a specialist sexual health service catering to urban clientele. Testing at this service is performed by dedicated technicians at their in-house laboratory using a high-volume throughput platform (GeneXpert Infinity) rather than by clinical staff in a primary care clinic setting using a 4-module platform. Similar to the TTANGO program, test results are electronically returned to patient records through a bespoke, tailored connectivity system allowing seamless recording and distribution of results as required.

Molecular STI POC testing has recently been demonstrated to improve clinical outcomes in studies undertaken in Papua New Guinea, South Africa and Rwanda, but all these reported studies were of short-term duration (less than 1 year) [33–37].

From 2018 to 2023, the World Health Organisation also conducted a multi-country validation study which focused solely on the analytical performance of these POC tests on the same technology as that used in TTANGO [2, 3].

To our knowledge, there are no other examples globally of large, networked, decentralised molecular POC testing networks for STIs implemented and integrated in primary care settings, and with testing performed by clinical staff.

5.2 TTANGO provides a potential template for translation to low- and middle-income countries

The TTANGO STI POC Testing Program for chlamydia (as well as gonorrhoea and trichomoniasis) provides a perfect template on how to translate a POC testing model from a seed concept to an impactful national public health program embedded

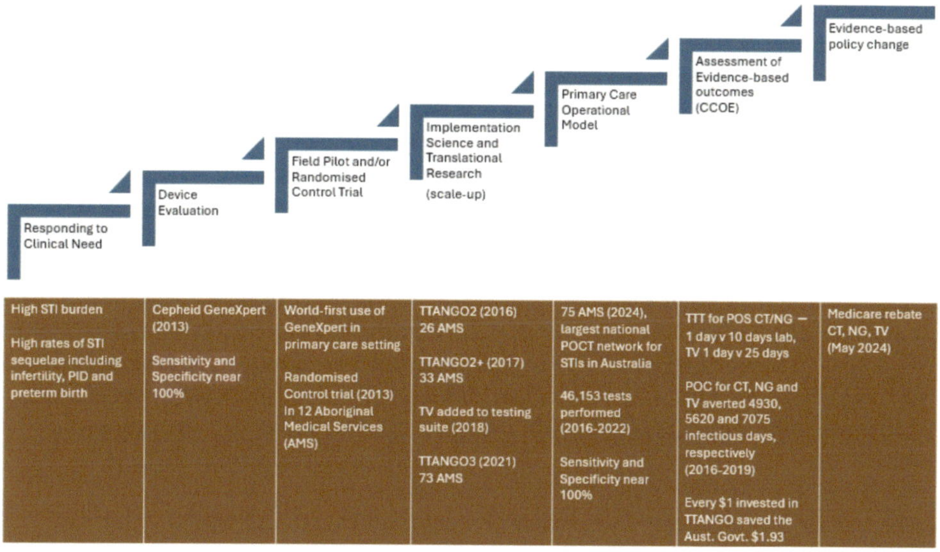

Figure 8.
From medical science to public health impact—the TTANGO Program.

in routine patient care (**Figure 8**). Using a systematic and stepwise research strategy over a decade in the making, the TTANGO network now represents a long-standing, sustainable and optimised network that could become a model for translation to low-and-middle income countries (LMIC) where *Chlamydia trachomatis* remains a significant contemporary health problem.

5.3 Challenges to translating this model to low- and middle-income countries

As mentioned previously, molecular STI POC testing has been trialled in several low-and middle-income health care settings including PNG, South Africa and Rwanda; however, this technology has not been widely scaled up in these settings [33–37]. While the affordability of the technology itself is often considered to be out of reach for low- and middle-income countries considering scale up of molecular technology, it is likely that the key infrastructure components will be the larger challenge to the translation of such a large, decentralised model in these settings. The need for a reliable power supply, dispersed connectivity, and secure supply chain for consumables, along with providing timely support for equipment maintenance and replacement to minimise disruption to use, are critical and rely on existing infrastructure. Ensuring a sufficient, competent cadre of POC test operators and the ability to offer ongoing support and troubleshooting to those as required needs to be tailored to the local setting. High turnover and limited workforce capacity is an issue often common to both high and low resource settings. A sustainable funding model to support the required infrastructure and operational implementation needs to be identified and confirmed in order to adequately scale up this model and ensure equitable access.

5.4 Challenges for the continuing evolution of the TTANGO program

While acknowledging the longevity and transferability of the TTANGO model, the TTANGO research team remains committed to investigate further means to continually improve the quality and scope of the program. Sources of sustainable funding need to be continually explored. To ensure equitable access and benefits of POC testing are available to all young people living in remote Australia, more work needs to be done to enhance POC testing uptake through collaborative, co-designed approaches including patient and provider engagement, alternative workforce models and POC testing integration as additional assays become available and expanded.

Key to the success of the TTANGO program is the ongoing active involvement of First Nations peoples and ACCHOs in all aspects of the program from its inception. STIs remain a sensitive area of healthcare, particularly in remote communities, and ensuring cultural safety for patients is a key consideration. Reducing shame and stigma associated with STIs, normalising STI testing and maintaining confidentiality are critical components to any STI program, particularly in small communities where healthcare workers may be related to their patients. While rapid test results enable faster access to treatment and contact tracing, consideration of who can access results, and how results are managed, must be prioritised to ensure patient safety.

As it has been demonstrated that the implementation of a decentralised STI POC testing program in regional and remote settings in Australia is feasible, acceptable, clinically effective and cost effective, there is an ethical imperative to ensure the technology is widely available in these settings. Currently the Medicare rebate for STI POC testing is only available to services in remote and very remote areas and yet a far higher proportion of First Nations peoples live in regional Australia. Therefore, the rebate should be extended to include these areas also to ensure equitable and sustainable access to STI POCT.

5.5 Future directions and emerging technologies for molecular-based POC testing

The GeneXpert system is comparatively expensive, technically complex and requires a laptop to drive the testing process. Consistent with the well-accepted REASSURED diagnostic criteria [14], global manufacturers should be continually encouraged to improve the affordability, accessibility and accuracy of future molecular-based technologies, as well as to provide devices with smaller footprints and assay methods with reduced turnaround time for results [14].

There is some light on the horizon. mobiNAAT is a mobile phone–based NAAT that uses a small magnetofluidic cartridge to perform isothermal amplification and provides results in around 1 hour. A small pilot of this technology measuring *Chlamydia trachomatis* was recently conducted in the emergency department setting and demonstrated 100% concordance with a laboratory NAAT [38].

The combination of CRISPR (clustered regularly interspaced short palindromic repeats) technology with isothermal amplification provides a novel means by which higher amplification efficiency of molecular targets and reduced reaction times can be potentially achieved on a less expensive and more user-friendly platform [39, 40]; indeed, CRISPR-based methods could become the new reality in the field of molecular diagnostics for infectious diseases over the next decade [41].

Acknowledgements

This book chapter is written on behalf of the large, multidisciplinary POC testing teams at the Flinders University International Centre for Point-of-Care Testing and the Kirby Institute. The authors acknowledge and thank the Australian Government

Department of Health and Aged Care for their support in funding the TTANGO POC Testing network. The authors acknowledge the contribution to these networks of many stakeholders including the participating aboriginal community controlled and government health services; jurisdictional and local aboriginal community controlled health organisations; state and territory health departments, and other government services; our industry and academic partners; pathology providers and most importantly, the dedicated health professional staff working as POC testing operators in the TTANGO network.

Conflict of interest

The authors have no conflict of interest to declare.

Author details

Mark Shephard[1*], Susan Matthews[1], Kelly Andrewartha[1], Gabi Hewer[1], Kirsty Smith[2], Louise Causer[2] and Rebecca Guy[2]

1 International Centre for Point-of-Care Testing, Flinders University, Adelaide, Australia

2 Kirby Institute, University of New South Wales, Sydney, Australia

*Address all correspondence to: mark.shephard@flinders.edu.au

References

[1] World Health Organization. Chlamydia fact sheet. 2023. Available from: https://www.who.int/news-room/fact-sheets/detail/chlamydia# [Accessed: September 03, 2024]

[2] Shephard M, Matthews S, Andrewartha K, Dimich W, Cabuang L, Barbara C, et al. Quality control and external quality assessment for the independent clinic-based evaluation of point-of-care testing to detect *Chlamydia trachomatis*, *Neisseria gonorrhoeae* and *Trichomonas vaginalis* in eight countries. BMC Infectious Diseases. 2024;**24**(Supplement. 1):Article 203. DOI: 10.1186/s12879-024-09057-x

[3] Shephard M, Matthews S, Kularatne R, Andrewartha K, Blondel K, Alvarez C, et al. Independent clinic-based evaluation of point-of-care testing for the screening of *Chlamydia trachomatis*, *Neisseria gonorrhoea* and *Trichomonas vaginalis* in women-at-risk in Australia, Guatemala, Morocco, and South Africa. BMC Infectious Diseases. 2024;**24**(Supplement. 1):Article 277. DOI: 10.1186/s12879-024-09018-4

[4] Morgan J, Colonne C, Bell A. Trends of reported chlamydia infections and related complications in New Zealand, 1998-2008. Sexual Health. 2011;**8**:412-418. DOI: 10.1071/SH10101

[5] Causer L, Liu B, Watts C, McManus H, Donovan B, Ward J, et al. Hospitalisations for pelvic inflammatory disease in young aboriginal women living in remote Australia: The role of chlamydia and gonorrhoea. Sexually Transmitted Infections. 2022;**2022**(**98**):445-447. DOI: 10.1136/sextrans-2021-055242

[6] Guy R, Ward J, Wand H, et al. Coinfection with *Chlamydia trachomatis, Neisseria gonorrhoeae* and *Trichomonas vaginalis*: A cross-sectional analysis of positivity and risk factors in remote aboriginal communities. Sexually Transmitted Infections. 2015;**91**:201-206. DOI: 10.1136/sextrans-2014-051535

[7] Natoli N, Causer L, Motta L, Shephard M, Guy R. Point-of-carc testing for chlamydia, gonorrhoea and trichomoniasis. In: Shephard M, editor. A Practical Guide to Global Point-of-Care Testing. Melbourne, Australia: CSIRO Publishing; 2016. pp. 378-392

[8] Hengel B, Wand H, Ward J, et al. Patient, staffing and health Centre factors associated with annual testing for sexually transmissible infections om in remote primary health centres. Sexual Health. 2017;**14**:274-271. DOI: 10.1071/SH16123

[9] Spaeth BA, Shephard MDS, Schatz S. Point-of-care testing for haemoglobin A1c in remote Australian indigenous communities improves timeliness of diabetes care. Rural and Remote Health. 2014;**14**:2849. Available from: http://www.rrh.org.au/articles/printviewnew.asp?ArticleID=2849

[10] Shephard M, Matthews S, Markus C, de Courcy-Ireland, Duckworth L, Haklar I, et al. Pathology testing at the point of patient care: Transformational change for rural communities. In: Rusangwa C, editor. Rural Health - Investment, Research and Implications. London, UK: IntechOpen; 2023. pp. 1-29. DOI: 10.5772/intechopen.109769

[11] Shephard M, Matthews S, Causer L, Hengel B, Guy R. Point-of-care testing in rural and remote Australia – An emerging technology to address global health challenges, crises and

security. In: Michaud A, editor. Global Health Security – Contemporary Considerations and Developments. London, UK: IntechOpen; 2023. pp. 1-23. DOI: 10.5772/intechopen.113849

[12] Shephard M, Shephard A, Matthews S, Andrewartha K. The benefits and challenges of point-of-care testing in rural and remote primary care settings in Australia. Archives of Pathology and Laboratory Medicine. 2020;**144**(11):1372-1380. DOI: 10.5858/arpa.2020-0105-RA

[13] Shephard M. Principles of establishing and managing a point-of-care testing service. In: Shephard M, editor. A Practical Guide to Global Point-of-Care Testing. Melbourne, Australia: CSIRO Publishing; 2016. pp. 16-28

[14] Land K, Boeras D, Chen X-S, Ramsay A, Peeling R. REASSURED diagnostics to inform disease control strategies, strengthen health systems and improve health outcomes. Nature Microbiology. 2019;**4**:46-54. DOI: 10.1038/s41564-018-0295-3

[15] Spaeth B, Matthews S, Shephard M. Patient-centred point-of-care testing: A life-changing technology for remote health care. In: Onal A, editor. Primary Health Care. London, UK: IntechOpen; 2021. pp. 1-15. DOI: 10.5772/intechopen.100375

[16] Spaeth BA, Kaambwa B, Shephard MDS, Omond R. Economic evaluation of point-of-care testing in the remote primary health care setting of Australia's Northern Territory. ClinicoEconomics and Outcomes Research. 2018;**10**:269-277. DOI: 10.2147/CEOR.S160291

[17] Nous Group. Department of Health and Aged Care. Evaluation of COVID-19 point-of-care testing in remote and First Nations communities. 21 December 2022. Available from: https://www.health.gov.au/sites/default/files/2023-05/evaluation-of-covid-19-point-of-care-testing-in-remote-and-first-nations-communities_0.pdf [Accessed: August 26, 2024]

[18] Tabrizi SN, Unemo M, Golparian D, Twin J, Limnios E, Lahra M, et al. Analytical evaluation of GeneXpert CT/NG, the first genetic point-of-care assay for simultaneous detection of *Neisseria gonorrhoeae* and *Chlamydia trachomatis*. Journal of Clinical Microbiology. 2013;**51**:1945-1947. DOI: 10.1128/JCM.00806-13

[19] Causer LM, Guy RJ, Tabrizi SN, Whiley DM, Speers DJ, Ward J, et al. Molecular test for chlamydia and gonorrhoea used at point of care in remote primary healthcare settings: A diagnostic test evaluation. Sexually Transmitted Infections. 2018;**94**:340-345. DOI: 10.1136/sextrans-2017-053443

[20] Guy RJ, Ward J, Causer LM, Natoli L, Badman SG, Tangey A, et al. Molecular point-of-care testing for chlamydia and gonorrhoea among Indigenous people attending primary health services: A cross-over cluster randomised controlled trial. Lancet Infectious Diseases. 2018;**18**:1117-1126. DOI: 10.1016/S1473-3099(18)30429-8

[21] Natoli L, Guy R, Shephard N, Causer L, Badman S, Hengel B, et al. "I do feel like a scientist at times": A qualitative study of the acceptability of molecular point-of-care testing for chlamydia and gonorrhoea to primary care professionals in a remote high STI burden setting. PLoS One. 2015;**10**(12):Article e0145993. DOI: 10.1371/journal.pone.0145993

[22] Badman SG, Causer LM, Guy R, Tabrizi SN, Francis F, Donovan B, et al. A preliminary evaluation of a new

GeneXpert (Gx) molecular point-of-care test for the detection of *Trichomonas vaginalis*. Sexually Transmitted Infections. 2016;**92**(5):350-352. DOI: 10.1136/sextrans-2015-052384

[23] Badman SG, Causer LM, Guy R, Wand H, Donovan B, Tabrizi S, et al. A reliable and easy to transport quality control method for chlamydia and gonorrhoea molecular point of care testing. Pathology. 2018;**50**:317-321. DOI: 10.1016/j.pathol.2017.09.012

[24] Saha A, Andrewartha K, Badman S, Tangey A, Smith K, Sandler S, et al. A flexible and innovative connectivity solution to support national decentralised infectious diseases point-of-care testing programs in primary health services in Australia. Journal of Medical Internet Research. 2023;**25**(1):Article e46701. DOI: 10.2196/4670

[25] Causer L, Ward J, Smith K, Saha A, Andrewartha K, Wand H, et al. Clinical effectiveness and analytical quality of a national point-of-care testing network for sexually transmitted infections integrated into rural and remote primary care clinics in Australia, 2016-2022: An observational program evaluation. The Lancet Regional Health – Western Pacific. 2024;**48**:101110. DOI: 10.1016/j.lanwpc.2024.101110

[26] Lafferty L, Smith K, Causer L, Andrewartha K, Whiley D, Badman S, et al. Scaling up sexually transmissible infections point-of-care testing in remote aboriginal and Torres Strait islander communities: Healthcare workers' perceptions of the barriers and facilitators. Implementation Science Communications. 2021;**2**(1):Article 127. DOI: 10.1186/s43058-021-00232-8

[27] Watts C, Causer L, Donovan B, Hui B, Tangey A, Smith K et al. The cost-effectiveness of molecular point of care testing for chlamydia, gonorrhoea and trichomonas in remote primary care health services in Australia. Presented at the 25th IUSTI World Congress; 17-20 September 2024; Sydney, Australia

[28] Wang S, Gum D, Merlin T. Comparing the ICERs in medicine reimbursement submissions to NICE and PBAC-does the presence of an explicit threshold affect the ICER proposed? Value in Health. 2018;**21**(8):938-943. DOI: 10.1016/j.jval.2018.01.017

[29] Hengel B, Causer L, Matthews S, Smith K, Andrewartha K, Badman S, et al. A decentralised point-of-care testing model to address inequities in the COVID-19 response. The Lancet Infectious Diseases. 2020;**21**(7):e183-e190. DOI: 10.1016/S1473-3099(20)30859-8

[30] Hengel B, Guy R, Casey D, Lorraine A, Smith K, Andrewartha K, et al. Decentralised molecular COVID-19 point of care testing: Contributions to the public health response and lessons learnt from implementing a primary care-based network in remote Australian communities. Medical Journal of Australia. 2024 (accepted for publication – Reference Number MJA23.01172)

[31] Modified Monash Model classification system for geographic remoteness. 2019. Available from: https://www.health.gov.au/sites/default/files/documents/2020/07/modified-monash-model-fact-sheet.pdf [Accessed: 8 September, 2024]

[32] Whitlock GG, Gibbons DC, Longford N, Harvey MJ, McOwan A, Adams EJ. Rapid testing and treatment for sexually transmitted infections improve patient care and yield public health benefits. International Journal of STD & AIDS. 2018;**29**(5):474-482. DOI: 10.1177/0956462417736431

[33] Badman SG, Vallely LM, Toliman P, Kariwiga G, Lote B, Pomat W, et al. A novel point-of-care testing strategy for sexually transmitted infections among pregnant women in high-burden settings: Results of a feasibility study in Papua New Guinea. BMC Infectious Diseases. 2016;**16**(1):250. DOI: 10.1186/s12879-016-1573-4

[34] Riddell MA, Vallely LM, Mengi A, Badman SG, Low N, Wand H, et al. Point-of-care testing and treatment of sexually transmitted and genital infections to improve birth outcomes in high-burden, low-resource settings (WANTAIM): A pragmatic cluster randomised crossover trial in Papua New Guinea. Lancet Global Health. 2024;**12**(4):e641-e651. DOI: 10.1016/S2214-109X(24)00004-4

[35] Garrett N, Mitchev N, Osman F, Naidoo J, Dorward J, Singh R, et al. Diagnostic accuracy of the Xpert CT/NG and OSOM Trichomonas rapid assays for point-of-care STI testing among young women in South Africa: A cross-sectional study. BMJ Open. 2019;**9**(2):e026888. DOI: 10.1136/bmjopen-2018-026888

[36] Mudau M, Peters RP, De Vos L, et al. High prevalence of asymptomatic sexually transmitted infections among human immunodeficiency virus-infected pregnant women in a low-income South African community. International Journal of STD and AIDS. 2018;**29**(4):324-333. DOI: 10.1177/0956462417724908

[37] Verwijs MC, Agaba SK, Sumanyi J-C, Umulisa MM, Mwambarangwe L, Musengamana V, et al. Targeted point-of-care testing compared with syndromic management of urogenital infections in women (WISH): A cross-sectional screening and diagnostic accuracy study. Lancet Infectious Diseases. 2019;**19**(6):658-669. DOI: 10.1016/S1473-3099(18)30724-2

[38] Shin DJ, Athamanolap P, Chen L, Hardick J, Lewis M, Hsieh YH, et al. Mobile nucleic acid amplification testing (mobiNAAT) for *Chlamydia trachomatis* screening in hospital emergency department settings. Scientific Reports. 2017;**7**:4495. DOI: 10.1038/s41598-017-04781-8

[39] Zhang L, Jiang H, Zhu Z, Lui J, Li B. Integrating CRISP/Cas within isothermal amplification for point-of-care assay of nucleic acid. Talanta. 2022;**243**:123388. DOI: 10.1016/j.talanta.2022.123388

[40] Luo H, Zeng L, Yin X, Pan Y, Yang J, Liu M, et al. An isothermal CRISPR-based diagnostic assay for *Neisseria gonorrhoeae* and *Chlamydia trachomatis* detection. Clinical. Microbiology Spectrum. Dec 2023;**11**(6):e0046423. DOI: 10.1128/spectrum.00464-23. Epub 2023 Oct 26

[41] Kostyusheva A, Brezgin S, Babin Y, Vasilyera I, Glebe D, Kostyusheva D, et al. CRISPR-Cas systems for diagnosing infectious diseases. Methods. 2022;**203**:431-436. DOI: 10.1016/j.ymeth.2021.04.007